CONTENTS

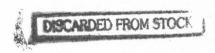

DISCARDED FROM STOCK

06188757

STAFFORDSHIRE
UNIVERSITY
LIBRARY

AGEING
TODAY

a positive approach to caring
for elderly people

VERONICA WINDMILL

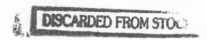

DISCARDED FROM STOCK

Edward Arnold

A member of the Headline Group

LONDON   MELBOURNE   AUCKLAND

Book No.   06188757

30121 0 06188757

STAFFORDSHIRE
UNIVERSITY
LIBRARY

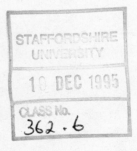

STAFFORDSHIRE
UNIVERSITY

10 DEC 1995

CLASS No.
362.6

Edward Arnold is a division of Hodder Headline PLC
338 Euston Road, London NW1 3BH

© 1990 Veronica Windmill

First published in the United Kingdom 1990

All rights reserved. No part of this publication may be reproduced
or transmitted in any form or by any means, electronically or
mechanically, including photocopying, recording or any information storage or retrieval system, without either prior permission in
writing from the publisher or a licence permitting restricted copy-
ing. In the United Kingdom such licences are issued by the
Copyright Licensing Agency: 90 Tottenham Court Road, London
W1P 9HE.

While the advice and information in this book is believed to be
true and accurate at the time of going to press, neither the author
nor the publisher can accept any legal responsibility for any errors
or omissions that may be made.

British Library Cataloguing in Publication Data
Windmill, Veronica
Ageing today: an approach to caring for the elderly
1. Old persons. Care
I. Title
362.6

ISBN 0-7131-8534-1

4 6 8 7 5 3
94 96 98 97 95

Typeset in 10/11 Baskerville by
Colset Private Ltd, Singapore
Printed and bound in the United Kingdom by
Athenaeum Press Ltd, Gateshead, Tyne & Wear.

INTRODUCTION

The process of ageing is very gradual and passes almost unnoticed by us all. Usually we only become aware of our increasing years by other people's reactions to us. Society tends to put limitations on us depending on our age and, for instance, we may be told 'you're too old to wear that/to go to dance class/to take up jogging' and so on.

Society's attitudes to ageing can help to create the idea that old age is a hopeless condition. In the West, the elderly are undervalued and often regarded as a burden because they are not given a valuable role to play. The enforced retirement age (65 for men and 60 for women) means that many elderly men and women feel useless and not respected. However, in the so-called less developed countries, the elderly tend to be respected for their wisdom and experience and are included in the extended family and given a useful role to play looking after the home and grandchildren while the parents work. Care of the elderly outside the family is virtually nonexistent. Until recently, jobs in caring for the elderly were less popular than other areas of caring. This attitude seems to be reflected in the prejudices that are held towards ageing.

- Many jobs, particularly those involving training, are closed to people over a certain age (often as young as 28!).
- Advertising tends to use young and attractive people to sell products and is geared towards a young audience.
- The elderly are less likely to receive certain medical treatments such as organ transplants and hip replacements than a younger person. There is often a general attitude that there is little point in treating conditions that are probably due to age.
- Stereotypes of the elderly, i.e., they are stubborn, foolish, forgetful and so on, are created and believed.

Ageism is the notion that people cease to be people, cease to be the same people or become of a distinct and inferior kind, by virtue of having lived a specified number of years. The eighteenth-century French naturalist Georges Buffon said, 'to the philosopher, old age must be considered a prejudice'. Ageism is that prejudice. Like racism, which it resembles, it is based on fear, folklore and the hang-ups of a few unlovable people who propagate these. Like racism, it needs to be met by information, contradiction and, when necessary, confrontation. And the people who are being victimised have to stand up for themselves in order to put it down.

(From Comfort, A., *A Good Age*,
Mitchell Beazley, 1977, p. 35: revised edition
The Joy of Age, Pan, 1989)

The number of elderly people in society is increasing year by year. Over the past 80 years the number of people past retirement age has risen from 4.7% to 14.5% of the population. We will all experience dealing with old age at some stage in our lives: we will either work with the elderly, care for elderly relatives, or experience it for ourselves.

The more knowledge and awareness we have of what it is like to grow old, the more it will encourage us to question our attitudes to the elderly and the type of care we offer them. It is to be hoped that this book will go part of the way towards creating a positive approach to caring for the elderly.

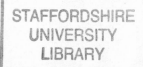
STAFFORDSHIRE
UNIVERSITY
LIBRARY

1
THE EFFECTS OF AGEING

Individuals age in different ways. Nowadays, old age tends to be defined by what a person can and cannot do, rather than by their chronological age. It is not unusual to see a spritely 80-year-old or, conversely, a 60-year-old who has become relatively disabled by old age. People of all ages are different and the elderly have a right to be seen as individuals with their own separate needs rather than bundled together as a faceless group.

How long we live and how healthy we are is determined by:

- our sex (women tend to live longer than men)
- our ethnic group (people in the West live longer than those in Third World countries)
- the medical and public health services available to us
- our environment
- our lifestyle
- factors inherited from our family background

Because people are tending to live longer old age may stretch over 30 years and there is obviously an enormous difference between the needs of a 60-year-old and those of a 95-year-old. These differences need to be taken into account when dealing with the elderly, and there is usually a distinction made between the young elderly (65–75) and the old elderly (75+) by medical and social workers. However, some generalisations need to be made about the ageing process, although it is stressed that these are only guidelines.

Physical changes affecting the elderly

Throughout life we lose nerve and body cells which are not replaced. This gradual degeneration of the body and nervous system causes the ageing process.

The most obvious signs of ageing are as follows.

- The skin loses its elasticity and becomes dry and wrinkled and brown patches of pigment appear.

- The hair loses its pigment and turns grey (although it is not unusual to find 20 and 30-year-olds who are grey). The hair becomes thin and dry as it loses its natural oils.
- Muscles shrink and waste away: this causes the elderly to lose their strength and agility and become tired more easily.
- Bones become brittle and are more likely to fracture because there is a reduction in the amount of calcium in the bones. Women suffer

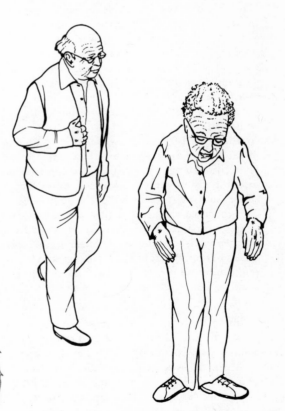

Fig. 1.1 Elderly people.

STAFFS UNIVERSITY LIBRARY

from this problem more than men because of various hormonal changes.

- The deterioration of the bones and muscles causes the elderly person to bend or stoop and to become up to 5 cm shorter.
- Muscle co-ordination and balance deteriorate.
- There is increasing difficulty in adjusting to extremes of heat and cold.
- The senses are affected. The sense of touch becomes less acute, so the elderly person may not respond to pain. Eyesight and hearing problems increase.
- The heart, being a muscle, becomes less efficient and less blood is pumped around the body with each beat, causing poor circulation and other problems.
- The lungs become less elastic and therefore take in a smaller amount of air, causing breathlessness. The lungs also become less efficient at removing oxygen from the air to keep the body functioning well which provides the elderly person with less energy and puts a strain on the heart.
- The digestive system, made up of a series of muscles, becomes less efficient. Food in the stomach is not adequately broken down by the muscles in the stomach wall, leaving much of the food undigested which may cause weight loss. The muscles in the gut wall lose elasticity and take longer to push the food along the alimentary canal, which is one of the possible causes of constipation.
- As the heart becomes less efficient at pumping blood around the body the rate at which blood flows through the kidneys is reduced to such an extent that waste products build up in the bloodstream and affect the health of the body cells.
- The menopause means that a woman can no longer reproduce. The hormonal changes during the menopause cause a loss of elasticity and lubrication in the vagina, breast shrinkage and loss of pubic hair. However, an older man can still father children, although he has fewer healthy sperm.

It is important to note that all these signs of ageing can develop into chronic health disorders, i.e., problems with the bones and joints may develop into arthritis, and a loss of the sense of touch may lead to hypothermia. People caring for the elderly, and the elderly themselves, need to be aware of the difference between what is an acceptable part of ageing and what is a potentially harmful disability or illness.

Health problems of the elderly will be dealt with in Chapter 3.

Mental changes affecting the elderly

A deterioration of the mental faculties is usually considered to be part and parcel of the ageing process. However, mental deterioration is frequently caused by anxiety, depression, lack of stimulation or low expectations. Research has found that if the elderly are offered too much help, their independence diminishes and they become more helpless and dependent and less able to cope mentally. Although certain mental powers reduce with age, any dramatic loss of mental powers should be investigated to find the cause.

The following are some of the acceptable mental changes in old age.

- Short-term memory loss (forgetting what has happened in the recent past) which is common in old age. However, the long-term memory can recall events of the distant past very clearly.
- Intellectual powers slow down; the elderly person does not become less intelligent, but will take longer to absorb new information.
- The personality may become more entrenched. The elderly tend to dislike change, but their inflexibility is usually because they can manage better and make fewer mistakes in their own surroundings.

As with the physical signs of ageing, any major changes should be investigated. A substantial loss of mental powers usually indicates an underlying mental health problem.

Social changes affecting the elderly

The elderly need to cope with the social effects of ageing, and come to terms with any changes; some may need help if the changes become insurmountable problems.

- Retirement, which may cause any combination of these four problems.
  - (i) Rejection because the person is no longer a useful member of society; loss of status.
  - (ii) Leaving the social life at work; loss of friends and colleagues.
  - (iii) Salary replaced by a pension; this usually causes a drop in living standards.
  - (iv) Additional leisure time without, perhaps, the money to finance leisure interests or

any other interests outside work; loss of direction.

- Loss of self-respect as the elderly person becomes increasingly dependent on family and professional agencies.
- Isolation leading to loneliness, even when amongst other people. The isolation may be caused by communication problems (sight or hearing defects), depression, grief, or living alone.
- Life changes, such as becoming grandparents or bereavement, making major demands on the elderly.

Summary of keypoints

- The ageing process is caused by a loss of body cells which make the body and nervous system gradually degenerate. This degeneration affects both mind and body.
- The social changes faced by the elderly may include retirement, an increasing dependence on family and professional agencies, loneliness, isolation and life changes such as bereavement.

Assignments

1. Find out about the factors affecting longevity (the length of life) by answering these questions.

- *Sex* What is the average life expectancy of men and women in Great Britain?

- *Ethnic group* Compare the life expectancy of men and women who live in the West with men and women who live in Third World countries.
- *Medical and public services* Make a list of the ways medical and public services help people to live longer.
- *Environment* What factors in our everyday lives may cause potentially fatal health problems?
- *Inherited factors* Make a list of diseases and disorders that we may inherit.

2. The number of people past the age of retirement is steadily increasing and people are living longer; this will put an even greater demand on the caring services which are already overstretched. Make a long-term plan for the care of the elderly using the following suggestions which may be helpful:

- likely changes in the pattern of the elderly population
- the potential needs of the elderly (social, physical, medical and emotional)
- responsibility for provision (local, national, voluntary, statutory)
- ways of improving society's attitude to the elderly
- the role of the carer
- education to prepare people for old age

3. The way a society regards ageing is reflected in the way its social policy provides for the elderly population. Compare the social policies of Great Britain with those of another country and evaluate the strengths and weaknesses.

STAFFS UNIVERSITY LIBRARY

2
SIGNS OF AGEING

Most living organisms have a set life span, and man is no different. The Bible sets our life span at three score years and ten (70 years), yet in this century many people in the West are living longer than this.

Ageing is a gradual yet natural process, the result of which is death; even healthy people must die. There are many theories that try to explain why we age. These theories include the idea that as each cell in our body reproduces itself it becomes less perfect each time which causes the body tissues to age. Another theory suggests that the protein present in the cells may alter and create less-efficient cells which again leads to ageing of the tissues. Finally, it has been suggested that our immune systems may become directed towards our own body cells and gradually destroy them. It is likely that ageing could be a combination of any of these theories plus our genetic make-up (what we inherit from our parents) our environment (where we live), what we eat, whether we exercise and so on.

Physical signs of ageing

1. The skin becomes dry and wrinkled for the following reasons:

- inherited factors
- hormone imbalance

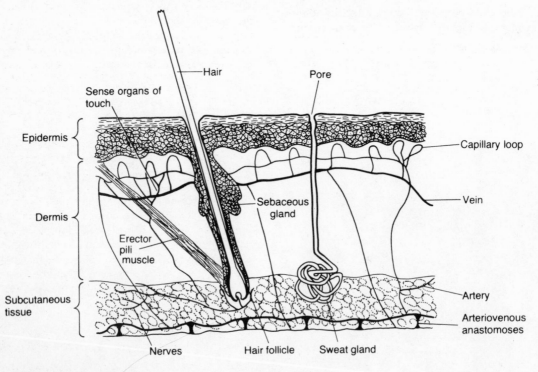

Fig. 2.1 A cross-section of the skin.

- thinning of the layer of fat below the skin's surface (subcutaneous fat)
- loss of elasticity as collagen levels are reduced
- a reduction in the number of sebum and sweat glands
- a reduction in the number of pigment cells

It is not possible to prevent wrinkles forming, but certain steps can be taken to slow down the process. The elderly should be advised to:

- not sunbathe for long periods and always wear sunscreen
- moisturise the skin
- eat a healthy diet
- exercise the face muscles

2.   The hair, which is regularly renewed throughout life, undergoes changes with age:

- the rate of growth slows down
- the rate of regrowth slows down, leading to gradual thinning, especially for men who may go bald
- there is a loss of pigmentation leading to all body hair going grey
- the hair becomes dry as the sebum glands in the scalp reduce in number and efficiency

Good hair care is beneficial and good for self-esteem and the ageing person should be encouraged to:

- wash hair frequently yet gently with a mild shampoo
- comb hair gently
- seek advice about any hair and scalp problems

3.   Long-sightedness (presbyopia) may develop as soon as the early 40s. People who have previously had good eyesight may now need reading glasses because of changes in the eye due to ageing, and those who have worn glasses because of short-sightedness (myopia) may need to wear bifocals. It also becomes increasingly difficult for the elderly to distinguish between certain colour hues, particularly blues and greens, and it takes longer for them to adjust between light and dark.

In order to keep the eyesight as accurate as possible with increasing years, the guidelines set out below should be followed:

- eyesight should be checked regularly
- rooms and staircases should be well lit
- professional advice should be sought about any change in vision as it may well be a sign of a medical problem

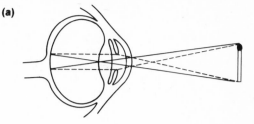

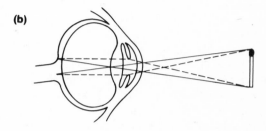

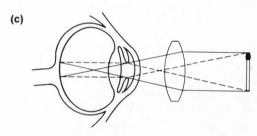

Fig. 2.2 (a) **Normal eyesight** The eye focuses on the matchstick and the image is projected upside down and back to front on the retina. The brain puts the image the right way up. (b) **Longsight (presbyopia)** The lens is less able to change shape so the image falls behind the retina. (c) **Corrective glasses** Opticians prescribe glasses with lenses that curve outwards making the image fall on to the retina.

4.   There will be gradual high frequency (high-pitched sounds) hearing loss after the age of 40, but this may not be noticed until many years later. The cause of this hearing loss is thought to be a loss of elasticity and a loss of hair cells in the inner ear, as these are both vital elements in transferring the sounds heard from the ear to the brain along the auditory nerve. Another type of hearing loss is due to one of the small bones in the middle ear fusing and not conveying the sound waves to the inner ear.

Hearing may be improved by having the ears syringed but, if the problem is untreatable, the person may be advised to wear one of the many types of hearing aids available. The following are some guidelines to help keep the ears as healthy as possible:

- hearing should be checked regularly and the ears syringed if necessary

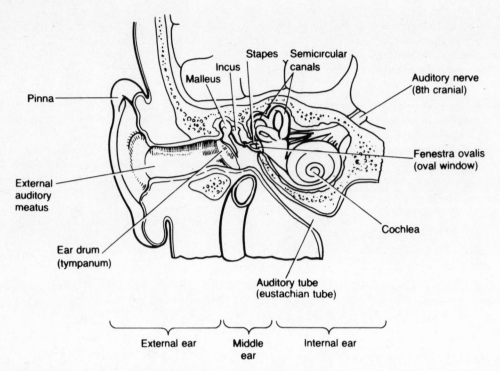

Fig. 2.3   The ear.

- assertiveness is required by those who need help with their hearing either by encouraging other people to use sign language, making sure that people speak clearly so that the person trying to hear and understand can lip read, or by asking people to lower their voice, rather than shouting, so that the low frequency sounds can be heard

5.   The ear is also the organ of balance and a deterioration in this function, coupled with a general weakness of the bones and muscles, leads to an increase in the number of falls in the elderly. Statistically, elderly women are twice as likely to fall as elderly men and are likely to suffer from broken wrists and hips as a result.

6.   The two senses of smell and taste are linked, and the elderly have an increasing difficulty recognising sweet and salty tastes. The elderly may tend to over season food to compensate, or may lose their appetites because of a lack of stimulation.

7.   Touch too may become less sensitive, and responsiveness to extremes of heat, cold and pain tends to be lost. There is the danger of the elderly not responding to cold and developing hypothermia, or failing to recognise that they are being burned by an overhot hot-water bottle or electric fire.

8.   The body composition (lean and fat ratios) alters with age and by the age of 40 the lean body mass (the parts of the body with no fat, i.e., the internal organs, muscles and bones) decreases and is replaced by fat. It is important that the elderly are aware of the dangers of putting on weight at this stage. Strength and stamina (the ability to keep going over a length of time) diminishes with age, even for people who exercise regularly, but particularly for those who do not. Fewer calories are needed per day in order to maintain weight. To avoid obesity in middle age regular exercise is needed and a reduction in the number of calories eaten.

9.   Healthy mouths and teeth are important, both for cosmetic and digestive reasons. Teeth need special care because, with increasing age, the following problems are likely to occur:

- gum disease which, if left untreated, will cause teeth to fall out
- badly fitting dentures because the elderly may not visit the dentist frequently enough
- changes in the jawline because of not wearing dentures or wearing badly-fitting dentures

Regular visits to the dentist should ensure that problems do not become long-term.

10. Legs and feet take a lot of wear and tear in everyday life and may need particular attention to help prevent problems developing. The following are some of the most common problems found in the legs and feet:

- poor circulation which may mean that minor injuries take longer to heal than usual; small sores that do not heal should be referred to a doctor to prevent them becoming infected
- corns and bunions
- chilblains
- ingrowing toenails
- skin diseases and ulcers
- varicose veins in the legs

The following guidelines may help to prevent the onset of foot and leg problems in old age:

- exercise should be taken to encourage blood circulation
- feet should be checked regularly for signs of problems and problems referred to a doctor or chiropodist
- feet should be washed daily and socks, stockings or tights changed
- toenails should be cut regularly, straight across
- baths should not be too hot
- good, well-fitting shoes which should grip the heel but not press the toes should be worn
- garters should not be used for keeping stockings up as they stop the blood circulating efficiently

11. Bones and muscles are affected by the ageing process and cause many problems if they are not functioning well. The average 70-year-old loses 5 cm in height because of a shortening of the bones in the back. The joints tend to enlarge, the bone mass shrinks and the muscle fibres reduce leading to many of the following problems:

- bad posture, which can be helped by regular exercise to prevent backache and loss of balance
- less strength, i.e., physical tasks take longer
- health problems because the muscles in the internal organs such as the heart, lungs and bladder are also affected

It is easy to assume that the symptoms of more serious ailments such as Parkinson's disease or arthritis (see p. 17) are part of the ageing process. However, any noticeable changes in physical ability should be referred to a doctor: *it is never normal for someone to be in pain.*

12. The digestive system is mainly governed by muscular actions and gland secretions, all of which are affected by the process of ageing.

- The muscles pushing the food along the digestive tract become weaker and less effective and the food takes longer to pass along the digestive system (see Fig. 3.4).
- The glands secreting gastric juices are less effective and produce few juices.
- Feelings of indigestion are noticeable.
- The gall bladder becomes less effective, causing more difficulty in digesting fats and a greater likelihood of developing gallstones or an inflamed gall bladder.
- Constipation is more likely as the muscles in the large intestine become less efficient.

Again, it is essential not to assume that the more serious digestive problems are just to be expected in old age. Any changes should be referred to a doctor. A healthy diet will, however, do much to help prevent minor digestive problems:

- foods high in fibre and nutritionally well-balanced should be eaten
- laxatives or other remedies should not be used without consulting a doctor
- rich and spicy foods should be avoided

13. The heart and blood vessels undergo various changes with age. The heart shrinks in size and the amount of fat surrounding it increases. Because the heart is a muscle it becomes less elastic and, therefore, less efficient and is not able to pump so much blood around the body with each beat. In most cases, enough blood will reach the body because the body needs less as the metabolism slows down. The heart is, however, less able to cope in times of stress. Because of the changes in the heart and blood vessels, plus hereditary and environmental factors, there is an increase in the incidence of high blood pressure in the West.

14. The respiratory system becomes less efficient with age: lung capacity shrinks and gaseous exchange (when oxygen is put into the bloodstream and carbon dioxide taken out) becomes less efficient. The elderly person therefore needs to breathe more during physical exertion in order to get enough oxygen. The elderly are more likely to be affected by respiratory disorders.

15. The urinary system becomes less efficient with age. The kidneys, which act as filters, become smaller and less able to filter out waste products effectively. This usually causes no problem but, if an

infection develops, the kidneys are less able to cope and are more likely to develop renal failure. Drinking about 1–1 ½ litres (2–3 pints) of fluid a day helps to keep the kidneys in good working order. In the elderly the bladder capacity reduces to roughly ¼ litre (½ pint), whereas a younger person's bladder holds over ½ litre (1 pint). The feeling of needing to pass water may be less noticeable and be the cause of slight incontinence. There are ways to help prevent problems in the urinary system:

- the bladder should be emptied frequently
- diuretics such as coffee and alcohol should be avoided
- if there are any unusual changes a doctor should be consulted
- plenty of fluids should be drunk

16.   Changes in the reproductive system affect men and women differently. Women become infertile after the menopause (when their periods and ovulation stop) at the average age of 50. There are four basic symptoms of the menopause:

- periods become irregular and eventually stop altogether
- hot flushes (when the skin gets hot and red)
- loss of vaginal lubrication
- night sweating

These symptoms are thought to be the result of hormone changes. Although they are not serious, they can affect sleep and sexual relationships. If necessary, discussion with a doctor can help these problems. The menopause also has a psychological effect on women and they may suffer from:

- depression
- mood swings
- loss of memory
- lack of self-confidence
- feelings of inadequacy

Men's fertility is not affected as dramatically as women's, although they do produce fewer healthy sperm, but they are more likely to suffer from sexual problems because their sexuality may be affected by, for example, loss of libido (sex drive) or impotence. The causes of these problems are usually:

- boredom in a relationship
- overindulgence in alcohol and food
- over-emphasis of career
- ill-health

17.   The nervous system, which governs the brain and nerves, is greatly affected by ageing. Brain weight decreases and the neurons (nerve cells which conduct messages to and from the brain and the spinal cord) which are lost are not replaced: the result is that reaction time becomes slower. The effects of these changes are:

- the five senses become less acute
- memory function is reduced
- the ability to co-ordinate body movements is reduced
- temperature regulation becomes less efficient

Psychological aspects of ageing

As well as the physical signs of ageing, there are psychological aspects too.

1.   A great deal of controversy exists over the effects of ageing on the personality. There is the general stereotyped idea that the elderly are stubborn and awkward, and there are the theories that the elderly become introverted and cut off from society in order to cope with the prospect of death. It is unlikely that any theory is completely correct: the elderly are ordinary people who have grown old and they therefore demonstrate the same range of personalities that can be found in the average population. Elderly people's personalities are unlikely to actually change, although certain aspects may become more entrenched. People who depended on others a great deal in their younger days will become the dependent elderly, and people who have always coped independently will probably continue to do so as far as possible into old age. The only generalisation that seems to be based on fact is that the elderly are less likely to take risks, probably because experience has taught them the likely outcome of their actions.

2.   In a society that regularly demonstrates the prejudice of ageism, there is a tendency to believe that intelligence and intellectual abilities decline as people grow older, although there is no reliable research to back up this claim. Most research uses a cross-section of society to test intelligence levels across the ages. The problem with this method is that the tests could well be comparing above average intelligence young people with average intelligence older people, and so on. The only reliable tests would be to test the same person regularly throughout their life, from youth to old age, and measure any changes in intelligence. Mental decline is often caused by mental or physical illness, which would obviously affect the results of any tests.

Reaction time does decline with age. There are two main causes for this: ill health and slower decision-making processes, although lack of practise could play a part in this decline. The elderly can be just as creative as the young, as can be seen by many famous elderly people in the arts, for example, Salvador Dali, Pablo Picasso, Pablo Casals and so on. Certain aspects of the memory alter: short-term memory loss does appear with age (the person finds it difficult to remember recent events) although long-term memory remains the same. This does not affect the person's ability to learn new information, although they may need to use different methods of learning to compensate for the slower reaction time and short-term memory loss.

Looking at the information, it seems that many assumptions are made about the decline in mental ability amongst the elderly in our society that detrimentally affects the way they are dealt with. Perhaps a wider understanding of their needs would promote better care provision.

In order to remain psychologically sound and stable, the elderly's needs are much the same as those of society in general:

- a healthy and balanced diet
- good housing and good surrounding environment
- an acceptable standard of living
- good health
- emotional security
- leisure interests
- socialising (meeting friends and family)

Sociological effects of ageing

1. These vary around the world: in Western societies old age is seen as meaning a time of enforced retirement from employment. We only have to look at the detrimental effect unemployment has on the population today (increased mental and physical ill health) to realise the effect it has on the elderly. In the past, and in Third World countries today, the elderly continued to work and were useful members of society which gave them a sense of worth. Enforced retirement tends to make the elderly feel useless, and many have expectations of poverty, dependence, free time with nothing useful to do, and loss of status and companionship. Pre-retirement courses and planning are necessary to try to avoid many of the pitfalls of retirement, and society needs to consider how to help make the change from full-time paid employment to full-time leisure. Some ideas could be:

- pre-retirement courses for all employees
- more flexible working hours and jobsharing
- financial planning for pensions, etc., at the start of working life
- post-retirement involvement in industry

2. This century has seen many changes in family life. These changes include:

- the increasing independence of women
- increasing mobility as families move to find employment
- broader and longer education for all children
- the size of families can be controlled by contraception

One of the results of these changes is that the elderly no longer need to take an involved role in grandparenting as they did when the extended family (three generations living under one roof – or living very close to each other) was more the norm. Today, families tend to be nuclear (parents and children living as one family) and mobile, so grandparents may live a long distance away from their children and grandchildren. This may not be a bad thing as many grandparents today have been used to living independently and do not want the added burden of regularly caring for grandchildren; they enjoy their company but value the freedom from ties. In the not too distant future, a greater number of the elderly will have no family as they have chosen not to have children themselves.

Problems may arise when a husband or wife dies and the remaining partner is left to cope with his/her grief and a dramatic change in lifestyle (see bereavement p. 40). The support of family and friends is vital at this time to help work through the various stages of grief, and prevent the tragedy of loneliness.

3. As the ageing person becomes more elderly they tend to lose much of their independence due to mental and physical decline and ill health. It can be difficult for various members of the family to cope with these role changes. For example, the child who used to look to the parent for help and support finds him/herself taking on the role of carer, whilst the ageing parent has to take on the role of dependent. In order to cope with these major changes, the elderly may become stubborn and unhelpful and the carer may feel resentful. These problems are just as likely to arise if the elderly person is cared for by the community. There are no easy answers to help cope with these problems, but the general beliefs that the elderly still have a right to be responsible for themselves as far as possible, and are still valued members of society, are vital when decisions are being made.

Summary of keypoints

- Ageing and death are natural processes.
- There is a difference between ageing and ill health: changes in the body causing pain or illness should be referred to a doctor.
- Personal care can help prevent health problems and regular check-ups can treat a problem before it becomes chronic.
- Regular exercise can help keep the body in good working order.
- Society's attitudes to ageing often mean the elderly have low expectations.
- Retirement should be given a more positive image and should not be regarded as the end of useful employment.
- The elderly deserve as much respect for their individual rights as the rest of society.

Assignments

1.   Preparation for the effects of ageing on the body should start early in life. Write a set of guidelines to help men and women prepare their bodies for the process of ageing. Include:

- skin
- hair
- eyes
- ears
- mouth and teeth
- body
- feet
- general appearance

2.   Many expensive cosmetic firms promote creams that can prevent the effects of ageing, get rid of wrinkles and so on. Look at some of the claims of the manufacturers and look at the ingredients in their products. Discuss whether you feel these claims are valid.

3.   In the past, the elderly were advised to eat rather bland foods such as steamed fish and stewed meats. What foods would you recommend a residential home to serve to their residents?

4.   Arrange a visit to a chiropodist's practice, or for a chiropodist to come and talk to your group, and find out about the work they do.

5.   Find out about exercise classes for the elderly in your area. These may be provided by the Community Education Department of the local schools and colleges, or by the Health or Social Services.

- Are there many classes?
- Do they reach any outlying areas?
- Are they well attended?
- What are the aims of the class tutors?
- Is there a fee?

6.   The ageing process is natural. Talk to friends and older members of your family about how it feels to grow older in terms of:

- physical changes
- psychological changes
- sociological changes

   Use your findings as the basis of a group discussion about any misconceptions you may have had about growing older.

7.   Compile a group survey to find out the attitude of the general public towards the elderly. You could include their attitudes towards:

- physical changes
- mental and intellectual abilities
- personality changes
- their role in society
- their role in the family
- the type of care provision they should have

   The answers you get may show some set ideas so be sure to note the age and sex of the people you interview. What conclusions do you reach about the results of your survey?

3

HEALTH PROBLEMS IN THE ELDERLY

In old age more mental and physical health disorders usually develop because the body gradually degenerates due to the ageing process and because life tends to be quite stressful around middle age. It is the physical and mental degenerative diseases that cause most of the problems as infectious diseases have, in the main, been eliminated by improved medical treatment. The major health problems in old age today are caused by:

- heart and circulatory diseases causing coronary heart disease (CHD) and strokes, often resulting in death
- cancer, which is usually fatal
- arthritis and other bone diseases which, although not fatal, are very painful
- brain disease leading to a loss of mental faculties and loss of independence

The common health disorders can either be treated or, if recognised early enough, at least made less debilitating. Sometimes it is difficult to recognise illness in the elderly, so a knowledge of what to look out for can be valuable.

Physical disorders

Urinary incontinence

Incontinence can range from mild to extreme:

- stress incontinence; urine may leak out when the person coughs, sneezes, laughs or exerts him/herself
- a dribbling of urine, for instance, in a man with a prostate problem
- an accident because the person cannot reach the toilet in time
- bladder infections
- the brain's failure to recognise the need to empty the bladder

The elderly person who suffers from incontinence needs to be medically examined to find out the cause of the problem. The next step is treatment or, if this is not possible, the incontinence needs to be dealt with as practically as possible. Dealing with incontinence is called continence management. Treatment may take the form of:

- antibiotics to cure infections
- exercises to strengthen pelvic floor muscles
- surgery to remedy prostate problems or strengthen pelvic floor muscles, etc.

There is, however, no cure for many of the causes of incontinence; the elderly suffering from mental deterioration can never be cured. In these cases, continence management can help cope with the problem. Urinary continence management involves discussion with the doctors and nurses dealing with the sufferer. Many health authorities run a continence advisory service. It is important that reversible incontinence is recognised and treatment recommended. Continence management may take any of the following forms.

- Habit reinforcement; the person's own patterns of urinating are observed and visits to the toilet made at these intervals in order to avoid accidents.
- Regular toileting, say every couple of hours, to prevent accidents. This form is used if the person's urinating patterns seem random.
- For men, a latex sheath attached to the penis collects urine in a small bag worn on the leg.
- Pads inserted into special pants, which need regular changing, are able to absorb urine and can be used for both men and women.
- Catheters inserted into the bladder may give the person mobility but need the full agreement of the individual to be used successfully. Catheters are more likely to cause bladder infections, but often their usefulness outweighs any problems.

STAFFS UNIVERSITY LIBRARY

When dealing with incontinence, the sufferer's self-respect needs to be considered: continence management should be indetectable by both eye and nose.

Faecal incontinence

This is a particularly distressing problem for the sufferer and for the people caring for him/her. Again, like urinary incontinence, if the problem cannot be treated, then it can be managed in a way that makes it easier for everyone concerned. The causes of faecal incontinence are:

- senile dementia
- constipation; the stools become hard and more difficult to pass and block the bowel so the faeces higher up become liquid in order to pass the blockage and they may leak out of the anus
- eating the wrong diet which may help to create excessively loose stools
- physiological problems such as cancer of the rectum, prolapse of the rectum, lesions and so on
- unexpected diarrhoea and an inability to reach the toilet

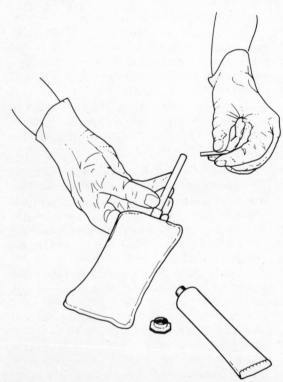

Fig. 3.1 Disposable enema **1**. The cap at the end of the nozzle is removed. **2**. Lubricating jelly is applied to the end of the nozzle. **3**. The nozzle is inserted up the rectum.

Once the medical and physiological problems have been treated, the sufferer may return to his/her normal bowel habits. Treatment may take the form of:

- removing the faecal blockage
- change of diet to prevent constipation/diarrhoea
- surgery

In cases where there is no hope of curing the problem, the person may need to wear padded pants.

Diseases of the heart and blood vessels

Heart disease

Heart disease is one of the major causes of death in the West. Fatty deposits (atherosclerosis) build up in the blood vessels and cause coronary heart disease and strokes. Some sufferers of heart disease may need amputations as the blood does not circulate through the body properly. The build-up of fatty tissue is associated with ageing, and a number of additional factors add to the problem:

- high cholesterol levels in the bloodstream, usually as a result of eating foods high in saturated animal fats
- high blood pressure
- smoking
- an unhealthy diet, high in fat, sugar and salt and too low in fibre
- inherited factors
- lifestyle (see below)

Except for inherited factors, we can make sure that the type of life we lead does not increase our chances of heart disease.

The heart may be affected by heart disease in four ways:

1. *Angina pectoris* This condition is caused by a temporary lack of blood supply to the heart. It causes severe but brief pains in the chest which may reach the arms, back, neck and/or jaw. It may be brought on by excess eating, smoking, physical exertion or emotional stress.

2. *Hypertension* (high blood pressure) If a person's blood pressure gets too high it can lead to coronary heart disease, brain disorders, kidney failure, arterial disease and strokes. The symptoms of raised blood pressure are dizziness, headaches, and a difficulty in concentrating and remembering. The condition may be caused by being overweight, eating a poor diet or a diet high in salt, stress or smoking.

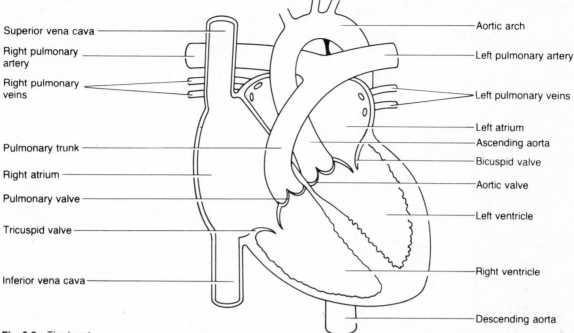

Superior vena cava

Right pulmonary artery

Right pulmonary veins

Pulmonary trunk

Right atrium

Pulmonary valve

Tricuspid valve

Inferior vena cava

Aortic arch

Left pulmonary artery

Left pulmonary veins

Left atrium

Ascending aorta

Bicuspid valve

Aortic valve

Left ventricle

Right ventricle

Descending aorta

Fig. 3.2 The heart.

The usual treatment is rest or drugs, although drug treatment is less successful in the older elderly person.

3. *Heart attack* This is when the blood supply is cut off from any part of the heart and the area then dies. Heart attacks may be mild and pass unnoticed, or they may be more severe and even fatal. The elderly may suffer a heart attack with little of the pain the middle aged may have, so any shortness of breath, pain or dizziness should be reported to a doctor as soon as possible. The causes of heart attacks may be a blocked artery to the heart, or a blood clot somewhere else in the body that upsets the heart beat. The majority of deaths due to heart attacks happen within minutes of the attack.

The treatment for heart attacks is:

- resuscitation, i.e., mouth-to-mouth and cardiac massage techniques
- coronary care units in hospital which provide life-support technology
- rest, preferably at home, as the surroundings are familiar and less traumatic

4. *Heart failure* Heart failure happens when the heart is unable to cope with the task of pumping blood around the body. This may be caused by high blood pressure, coronary heart disease, chest infection or general illness in the elderly person. In severe cases, the sufferer will be very breathless and develop a build-up of fluid in the lungs which will need treatment by diuretic drugs which get rid of the excess fluid as urine. In more chronic cases, the excess fluid will collect in the legs and milder forms of diuretics will be needed to clear up the problem.

Strokes

Strokes are caused by diseased blood vessels in the brain, usually found to be haemorrhages or blood clots, which starve the brain of oxygen (see Fig. 3.3). As with the heart, the area deprived of oxygen dies and the part of the body controlled by the dead area of the brain no longer functions. The part of the body affected will be on the opposite side of the brain to that which has suffered the stroke.

Strokes may take many forms, some mild and some severe, ranging from:

- a temporary interruption to the brain's blood supply which usually gets better within 24 hours. Symptoms of this form of stroke may be temporary blindness in one eye, or one side of the mouth may be paralysed
- a stroke which gets worse over a number of days
- a severe stroke affecting all the body causing total paralysis

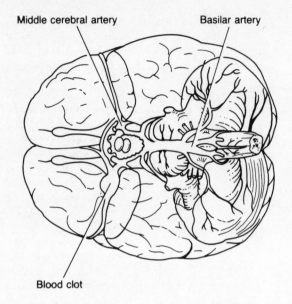

Middle cerebral artery   Basilar artery

Blood clot

Fig. 3.3 A stroke can be caused by a blood clot or a haemorrhage in the brain.

- paralysis of half the body (hemiplegia)
- paralysis of one arm or leg (monoplegia)
- unusual social behaviour such as confusion or disorientation
- slurred speech (dysarthria) or losing the ability to speak or understand speech (aphasia and dysphasia)

Strokes caused by a brain haemorrhage are usually more dangerous because the blood continues to leak into the brain causing more damage and the effects are immediate. Strokes caused by a blood clot usually come on more gradually and, although often leaving the person partially paralysed, respond better to therapy. It may take years to recover from a stroke and even then the victim may not return to complete normality. The victim will need plenty of help and support from family, friends and the community.

Circulatory problems

Circulatory problems in other parts of the body.

- It is possible for the arteries supplying blood to the legs to become blocked. Sometimes surgery may help to clear the blockage but if this is not possible then the leg will need to be amputated, usually below the knee.
- A blood clot may get into the larger veins in the leg, sometimes after an operation, and cause pain

and swelling. There is a danger that the clot may move on to the heart or lungs and prove fatal. Blood clots like this are usually treated by anti-coagulant drugs (drugs that prevent the blood from clotting).

Diseases of the respiratory system

The lungs of the elderly person are prone to various disorders because of a loss of resistance to bacterial infections. Unusual symptoms should not be assumed to be part of ageing but should be referred to a doctor.

- Pneumonia is fairly common in the elderly and it tends to strike those who are already suffering from other dangerous illnesses which may cause death. Infection of one lung is called lobar pneumonia and infection of both lungs is called bronchopneumonia. The symptoms of pneumonia are coughing, breathlessness, weakness and fever, and there may be some pain. It can be treated by antibiotics and physiotherapy, and most elderly people respond to treatment.
- Bronchitis may be either acute or chronic.
  Chronic bronchitis tends to be an ongoing disability and is usually caused by smoking or working in a dusty atmosphere. The symptoms are a cough, caused by an increase in mucus in the lungs, which may last for up to three months over the winter and recur every year. Other complications may develop if the sufferer's situation does not improve; the mucus may become infected, the air passage may get blocked by inflammation, and heart failure may result because of the strain on the heart.
  Acute bronchitis is when the airway rather than the lungs is affected, resulting in phlegm being produced and coughing occurring to clear the airway.
- Lung cancer is usually associated with smoking, and the symptoms may be a persistent cough, coughing up blood, shortness of breath, pain in the chest and weight loss. Often the disease is too well-established before it is discovered and the outlook for recovery is poor, although treatment can help reduce any pain.
- Emphysema occurs when the tiny air sacs (alveoli) in the lungs become distended which makes the alveoli walls thin and they eventually rupture causing a lack of elasticity in the lungs. Emphysema is usually a result of bronchitis and/or ageing tissues. The symptoms are breathlessness and blue lips, and there is no successful treatment. The sufferer may go on to develop

heart failure because of the added pressure on the heart.

Problems of the digestive system

In old age, problems associated with the digestive system increase but become more difficult to diagnose, although early diagnosis means a greater chance of recovery. The symptoms to look out for are:

- loss of appetite
- weight loss
- nausea and vomiting
- diarrhoea
- pain
- constipation
- change in pattern of bowel movements
- blood or mucus in the stools

The following are some of the more common digestive disorders associated with old age.

- Duodenal or gastric ulcers, which develop when the stomach or duodenum lining becomes ulcerated, cause less pain in the elderly than in the young. Symptoms may include loss of appetite, slight pain and a feeling of general illness. If left untreated, the ulcer may cause a haemorrhage or burst (perforate) allowing the contents of the stomach to pass into the abdominal cavity. Surgery is rarely necessary and ulcers can usually be treated with drugs. The person does need to avoid smoking, drinking alcohol or taking aspirin-based drugs.

- Gallstones cause a great deal of stomach pain. In early old age women are more likely to have gallstones than men, but by the age of 70 the likelihood of either sex developing them is equal. The symptoms are nausea, particularly after eating a greasy meal, pain below the ribs on the right-hand side and vomiting.

  Milder gallstones can be treated by drugs that gradually dissolve them, but more serious cases need to be operated on.

- Diverticulitis occurs when small parts of the intestinal lining (diverticula) protrude through the intestinal wall allowing faeces to collect leading to an infection in the intestinal wall which causes pain and bouts of diarrhoea and constipation. The best method of prevention and treatment is to eat a very high fibre diet.

- Fear of constipation used to be the obsession of many British people, and still is for many elderly people. It is not necessary to open the bowels every day if that is not the normal pattern. What is important is that bowel habits do not inexplicably alter, and that the stools are not small and hard, making them difficult to pass. Constipation, in the true sense, can be caused by a low fibre diet, certain drugs, overuse of laxatives in the past, an underactive thyroid or an obstruction in the bowel. Any changes in bowel habit should be referred to a doctor to check the cause.

- Diarrhoea can be caused by a short lasting stomach bug, as with the rest of the population. It may, however, be the result of diverticulosis, inflammatory conditions, certain drugs, a change in diet or stress. It should be referred to a doctor if the symptoms persist longer than 24 hours.

- Haemorrhoids (piles) are varicose veins around the anus. They are usually situated just inside the anus, but are likely to come out if they become enlarged. The usual cause of haemorrhoids is pushing hard stools out while constipated. If left untreated, the haemorrhoids may become itchy,

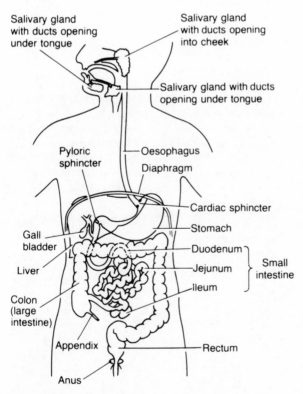

Salivary gland with ducts opening under tongue

Salivary gland with ducts opening into cheek

Salivary gland with ducts opening under tongue

Pyloric sphincter

Oesophagus

Diaphragm

Cardiac sphincter

Stomach

Gall bladder

Duodenum

Jejunum

Ileum

Small intestine

Liver

Colon (large intestine)

Appendix

Rectum

Anus

Fig. 3.4 The digestive system.

STAFFS UNIVERSITY LIBRARY

or bleed, leading to anaemia. Treatment may simply be creams and suppositories. If the condition does not improve, the haemorrhoids can be injected to shrink them, or surgically removed.

- Cirrhosis of the liver is untreatable and fatal. Cirrhosis may be caused by:

  - alcohol abuse (the most common)
  - damage from some drugs and chemicals
  - hepatitis B

The liver cannot be cured, although eliminating alcohol, if that is the cause, can prevent further damage. If left untreated, cirrhosis may also cause cancer or haemorrhaging.

Problems in the eyes

Change in vision is to be expected as we grow older, but there are other more serious disorders that may affect the eyesight of the elderly.

- Cataracts are very common in old age, and occur when the lens becomes clouded which prevents light reaching the retina. It is possible to operate to remove the cataract if vision becomes badly affected.
- Glaucoma occurs when pressure from the fluid in the eye builds up. The first symptoms may be poor vision, a pain in the eye, headaches and

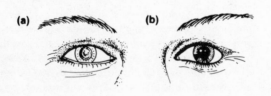

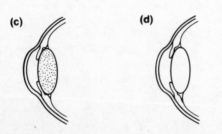

Fig. 3.5 The eye – with and without cataract **(a)** White pupil. **(b)** Normal eye. **(c)** Cataract in lens. **(d)** Lens.

nausea. If left untreated, glaucoma causes tunnel vision, i.e., when only things directly in front can be seen. There are two types of glaucoma:

(i) acute glaucoma is more sudden and needs surgery to remove part of the iris to stop the build-up of pressure

(ii) chronic glaucoma is more gradual and can be treated by eyedrops which reduce the secretions into the eye

Frequent eye check-ups are essential to detect signs of glaucoma as early as possible so that effective treatment can be started.

- The most common cause of blindness in the UK is diabetes which may cause either cataracts, destruction of the retina or glaucoma. In diabetics, new blood vessels are formed in the eye which destroy the retina and lead to loss of vision. These blood vessels can be treated by using lasers.

Problems in the mouth

On page 6 it was found that many elderly people suffer from gum disease and this is the major cause of loss of teeth. If there are some healthy teeth, dentists tend to leave them in as they give the mouth shape and also can be used to fix dentures to. Gone, hopefully, are the days when many elderly people went to the dentist and had every tooth taken out and had dentures fitted for convenience.

Although dentures have improved greatly, they can still cause problems. The danger is that the old elderly may not complain about their teeth but choose a soft diet instead which probably is not giving them all their nutritional needs and does not give their gums or salivary glands enough stimulation. It is important that dentures are correctly fitted and properly looked after. The following points should be considered when caring for the elderly who wear dentures:

- dentures may be poorly fitting because of gum shrinkage, and this will cause soreness and possible ulceration
- sets of dentures that bite together (occlude) badly will strain the jaws and cause pain and damage
- the mouth will collapse if poorly fitting dentures are worn. Taking care of dentures is quite simple if the basic guidelines below are followed

  (i) the dentist should be visited regularly to check that the dentures fit; the gums shrink a great deal for the first six months after dentures have been fitted and a top set of dentures will usually fit better than a lower set as the lower gums recede more

(ii) dentures should be thoroughly cleaned every day because, as well as being unhygienic, unclean dentures are as unpleasant as unclean teeth; dentures should be brushed with denture paste using a medium toothbrush, and the brushing should continue while the dentures are rinsed under the tap. Soaking dentures is fine for bleaching them and improving the whiteness, but it is not an effective way of removing food debris

(iii) dental fixatives are not usually worth using as they are not very effective

(iv) gums need to be kept in a healthy condition by cleaning them regularly with a mouthwash

Problems on the skin

As well as the usual signs of an ageing skin (p. 4) there are other problems which may develop as age increases.

- Warts, moles and spots tend to increase. Reddish spots (maculae) and brown warts develop on the body but neither of these are dangerous. Moles which increase in size or bleed should be referred to a doctor as they can be a symptom of skin cancer.
- Skin irritations may be the result of the dryness caused by ageing. Sometimes an infection may develop where folds of skin touch each other and have little air reaching them (inbetween the thighs, armpits, etc.). This sets up the right conditions for a fungus infection called intertrigo. Intertrigo can, however, be easily treated by using a fungicidal cream. Prevention is better than cure, however, and it can be avoided by not becoming overweight and increasing personal hygiene.
- Ulcerated legs are quite common in the elderly, especially on the ankles, and often affect people suffering from varicose veins. The ulcers are open, usually painless, sores and may be very small or up to several centimetres across. Fluid oozes from the ulcers and they are liable to become infected. Once infected they become very painful. If the ulcers are ignored they will last indefinitely but, if treated, they will usually clear up within a few weeks.
- Varicose veins on the legs may occur at any age, but often start in women during pregnancy. The

veins are raised and knotted and found on the lower leg. Because the veins stand out and have thin walls, there is a danger of damaging them and causing haemorrhaging. Sufferers will have a dull ache, especially if they have been standing for long periods of time, and will find it tiring to walk any distance. The causes of varicose veins are:

(i) jobs that involve a lot of standing

(ii) poor circulation in the legs

(iii) poor valves in the veins in the leg that allow the blood to pool in the lower leg

- Shingles (herpes zoster) is a very painful condition for the elderly. The herpes zoster virus is related to the chicken pox virus, so the elderly should avoid contact with children suffering from chicken pox. The symptoms of shingles start with a bad pain over an affected area of skin supplied by a nerve, a blistery rash then follows which lasts for 10–14 days and this is accompanied by a feeling of malaise. Shingles usually affects the chest area, but can also affect the head, face and eyes.

There is no treatment for shingles, but the pain of the symptoms can be helped by painkillers prescribed by a doctor and cool baths. If the shingles is caught at an early stage, antiviral drugs applied to the blisters can help reduce the pain. Complications can develop if shingles affects the eyes as this can cause blindness, so a doctor should always be informed.

Problems with the bones and joints

Walking is something people take for granted until something happens which makes movement painful. For many of the elderly with bone or joint disorders, loss of mobility is something that causes a great deal of pain and makes them unwilling dependents.

- Arthritis is the greatest cause of lack of mobility in the elderly. There are two forms of arthritis.

(i) *Osteoarthritis* is the more common, and it is a wearing down of the cartilage covering the ends of bones at the joints. Without the cartilage to make joint movements smoothe, there is a greater friction which can lead to inflammation and the muscles tend to become weaker. Osteoarthritis most commonly affects the joints which are most used, i.e., hips, knees, feet, hands and ankles. The symptoms are pain and swelling around the affected area. The cause of osteoarthritis is not really known, but it is thought to be a result of the ageing process and is not helped by being overweight, having bad posture or undergoing trauma to the joint (e.g., an accident, fall or sports injury, etc.). There is no cure for osteoarthritis, although it can be helped by anti-inflammatory drugs, pain-killers and physiotherapy which increases the muscle strength and helps with mobility.

If the hip is badly affected, the sufferer may have a hip replacement operation where an artificial hip made of metal and plastic is inserted in place of the damaged joint. The operation is becoming increasingly successful as artificial joints are being improved, although they do need to be replaced about every ten years.

(ii) *Rheumatoid arthritis* mainly affects the smaller joints such as the shoulders, ankles, toes, wrists, hands and fingers. It affects mainly women and can start at any age after about 25. Many elderly are, however, affected. It is less common than osteoarthritis but can be more crippling. Symptoms of rheumatoid arthritis are swollen joints, pain, stiffness and shiny, red skin over the affected joint. In time, the sufferer may lose weight, feel ill and feverish and lose their appetite. Anaemia may also develop along with other complications affecting the heart, lungs and kidneys. The cause of rheumatoid arthritis is also not known, although it is thought to be partly due to an allergic reaction. The disease goes through active phases and remission stages and after many years the phases may stop altogether, but the affected limbs will usually have been permanently damaged and deformed. It is treated by anti-inflammatory drugs and splinting of the limbs to protect them and help prevent deformity.

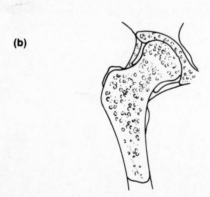

(a)

Cartilage

Lubricating fluid

Bone

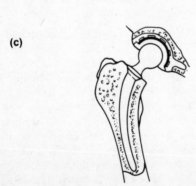

(b)

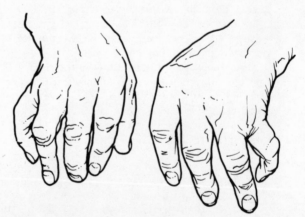

(c)

Fig. 3.6 Cartilage at the end of bone **(a)** Normal joint. **(b)** Damaged joint. **(c)** Artificial hip in position.

Fig. 3.7 Disfigured hands caused by arthritis.

Physiotherapy is vital because the problem will get worse if the joint is not used, although the sufferer does need to rest. During the remission phase the physiotherapist will recommend the correct exercising techniques to help improve the joints.

- Osteoporosis occurs when the bones weaken in old age because of a lack of calcium and protein. The problem occurs more in women than men and this is thought to be due to the effects of the menopause. The symptoms of osteoporosis are that bones break more easily and backache. The back may even curve, causing a height loss. Treatment is calcium and vitamin D supplements and physiotherapy, although regular exercise, especially after the menopause for women, is said to help prevent the problem developing.

- Osteomalacia may affect any age group, although it is more common in the elderly. It is similar to rickets and is caused by a lack of vitamin D which is needed to help absorb calcium. Again, it is more common in women than men. Treatment is vitamin D supplements and occasionally female sex hormones for women.

- Paget's disease mainly affects the elderly and is a thickening of the bones of the skull, spine, pelvis and legs. The bones thicken because the body stops the breakdown and reabsorption of the bone cells and this causes pain, frequent fracturing of the bones and a broadening of the skull. Complications arise if the affected parts become malignant. The cause of the disease is unknown, and it mainly affects people over the age of 40. Treatment for milder cases is painkillers and for the more painful cases hormone injections are given.

- Intermittent claudication is a very painful cramp that affects the legs when walking. It stops when the sufferer rests and comes on after walking a certain distance. It is caused by a restricted blood supply to the legs either because of diseased arteries or a blockage. If the disease gets worse, the foot may develop gangrene and need to be amputated. Treatment can be either to surgically remove the blockage or to operate on or inject the spine to increase the diameter of the blood vessels. Preventive treatment is to eat a healthy diet that will keep weight down and keep the bloodstream free of too much cholesterol, and to stop smoking.

- Falls, although not a disorder or disease, cause bruising and breakages and are the major cause of death in the elderly. There may be a number of reasons for falling:
  (i) loss of balance because of the ageing process, diseases of the inner ear, or a lack of blood supplied to the brain
  (ii) heart and circulatory disorders which affect the blood supply to the brain, e.g., high blood pressure, coronary thrombosis, heart palpitations and so on
  (iii) degenerative diseases affecting the limbs, e.g., Parkinson's disease, multiple sclerosis, etc.
  (iv) bone and joint disorders, e.g., osteoarthosis, arthritis, etc.
  (v) accidental falls such as tripping over
  (vi) drop attacks, when the elderly person suddenly falls to the ground for no apparent reason and there is a loss of the use of the legs; in order to get back on their feét the elderly person needs to put pressure on their feet again by, for example, pushing them against a wall

The problem with falls in the elderly is that the elderly lose self-confidence and may be less willing to go out in case they fall again and they may be unable to get help if they live alone. The other danger with falls is the development of hypothermia (see below) if the elderly person is left in the cold for any length of time.

Problems with the nervous system

With age, the nervous system becomes less effective at coping with messages from inside and outside the body.

1. *Hypothermia* is a well-publicised problem and occurs when the elderly person's body temperature drops below 95°C (35°F) because they are either ill, in cold surroundings, or their body temperature mechanism is not working properly. Hypothermia mainly affects the very old and feeble and those who are ill or too poor to heat their homes.

The symptoms of hypothermia are that the person feels cold to the touch and may be drowsy and confused. The heartbeat slows down and the muscles become stiff. Unconsciousness, brain damage and then death will occur unless action is taken. Hypothermia is treated by gradually warming up the person and their surroundings and getting them to hospital immediately. Warm drinks should not be

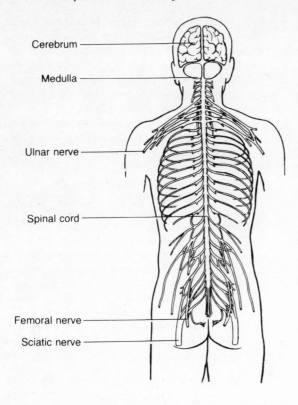

Cerebrum

Medulla

Ulnar nerve

Spinal cord

Femoral nerve

Sciatic nerve

Fig. 3.8 The human nervous system.

given because they divert the blood to the stomach. Prevention is the ideal so the elderly should be in warm surroundings with layers of light clothing to keep their body temperature comfortable.

2. *Multiple sclerosis* usually occurs between the age of 20–50, so the elderly with multiple sclerosis have usually had it for some time. Women develop this disease more often than men. The symptoms are blurred vision, feelings of heaviness or pins and needles in the limbs, bladder or bowel incontinence, change of mood, tremor in the arms and/or legs and lack of co-ordination. The disease is incurable, but physiotherapy can help the person stay independent for as long as possible. A spastic type of multiple sclerosis develops in the elderly where the muscles tighten into spasm and this may cause pain.

3. *Parkinson's disease* virtually only affects the elderly and causes muscular stiffness and tremor and affects more men than women. The first symptoms of the disease often pass unnoticed as the disease starts very gradually. Symptoms are tremors in the hands,

arms and legs that become worse as time goes on. The head may nod and the hands look as if they are rolling beads between the thumbs and fingers. Gradually the face muscles stiffen up and the expression becomes blank and staring, and the limbs become stiff and resistant to movement. As walking becomes more difficult, the sufferer stoops and shuffles. Depression is very common because the mind is unaffected and the person is aware of everything that is going on. In most cases the disease lasts for years, although it can cause death if the respiratory muscles are affected. There is no cure, but exercises and social interaction are valuable.

The physiotherapist and occupational therapist will give the sufferer exercises to improve mobility and muscle tone and a doctor can prescribe drugs to help relax the muscles. The medical profession has been looking for a cure to Parkinson's disease for years. At present surgeons are awaiting long-term results of controversial experimental operations where the brain cells from a dead foetus are injected into the brain of a person suffering from Parkinson's disease. As yet, there are no positive results.

4. *Motor neuron disease* occurs when the cell neurons of the motor nerves (those carrying messages from the nervous system to the muscles) are affected and certain muscles waste away. The disease most commonly affects the legs, hands, tongue or throat and the symptoms are wastage of the affected muscles and muscular twitching which is visible under the skin. The disease is incurable and if the throat is affected it can soon cause death as food tends to enter the lungs and cause choking or pneumonia. The cause of the disease is unknown, but some theories suggest it may be a virus infection.

5. *Subdural haematoma* is clotted or liquid blood that has collected in the subdural veins that run across the surface of the brain. A subdural haematoma may develop as the result of a head injury, even if the injury only seemed to be minor. The symptoms start days or weeks after the injury and may include headache, slowness, personality changes, confusion, fits and weakness on one side of the body. Once the problem has been diagnosed by X-ray or brain scan, the sufferer has a hole drilled through the skull to reduce the pressure on the brain. The success rate of treatment is reduced in the very old and frail elderly, especially if diagnosis has taken some time.

6. *Trigeminal neuralgia* is a very unpleasant condition. Brief but agonising pains are felt on one side of the lips, gums, cheeks or temples. The pains

may come in bouts and reappear again after weeks or even months and are very upsetting to the sufferer. Bouts of pain may be brought on by the cold, pressure, facial movements or a degeneration of the walls of blood vessels. Cases can be treated by painkillers or occasionally by injecting local anaesthetic into the nerve which provides relief for about two years.

7. *Brain failure* or *dementia* may have one or more contributory factors. There are two types of brain failure: acute, which starts suddenly, or the more gradual onset of chronic brain failure.

- Acute brain failure may show any combination of the following symptoms:
  - (i) serious confusion
  - (ii) hallucinations
  - (iii) delusions, e.g., suspicion and fears of persecution

  Acute brain failure usually has a physical cause which can often be treated. These causes include:
  - (i) infections
  - (ii) drugs
  - (iii) heart problems
  - (iv) metabolic disorders
  - (v) disorders of the nervous system, e.g., a stroke

  Once the problem has been diagnosed, treatment must be carefully planned as the shock of being admitted to a strange hospital may make the problems worse.

- Chronic brain failure starts gradually and becomes progressively worse. It affects all aspects of the brain, such as intelligence, personality and memory, and will also affect social and physical well-being. Many of the following symptoms will develop:
  - (i) loss of memory, starting with loss of short-term memory and then affecting the long-term memory
  - (ii) personality changes, including aggression and anti-social behaviour
  - (iii) general confusion about time, place and environment
  - (iv) loss of ability to concentrate
  - (v) self-neglect
  - (vi) tendency to wander and become disorientated
  - (vii) inability to cope with the problems of everyday life
  - (viii) apathy and unwillingness to move
  - (ix) incontinence
  - (x) inability to communicate with others, including close friends and family

Diagnosis of the condition is not always easy as the symptoms of brain failure may be confused with depression or lack of stimulation, both of which can be improved with correct diagnosis and treatment. Very occasionally, chronic brain failure may be the result of another physical, yet curable, disease such as an underactive thyroid, a brain tumour or vitamin deficiency. A brain scan will tell the doctor the cause of the elderly person's brain failure, but these scans are very expensive and are not generally available on the National Health Service.

There are two main causes of dementia.
  - (i) Alzheimer's disease, which accounts for roughly half of the chronic brain failure cases, occurs when the sufferer becomes progressively less able. The disease may run in families, although it is not necessarily genetically inherited, and may develop before the age of 60.
  - (ii) Multi-infarct disease occurs when areas of brain tissue die through lack of oxygen, usually as a result of strokes, high blood pressure and other cardiovascular problems.

Treatment of brain failure is difficult, except in the cases where there is an underlying cause. In general, treatment is limited to support from the domiciliary services (see p. 27), drugs to control sleeplessness, restlessness and aggressive tendencies, and liaison with social and health service workers to assess the patient's needs.

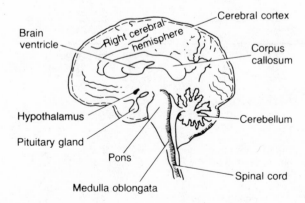

Fig. 3.9 Vertical section through the brain.

STAFFS UNIVERSITY LIBRARY

8.   *Depression* is a condition that can affect any age group, but the elderly are prone to depression as old age is often accompanied by loneliness, ill health, bereavement, lack of money and loss of status in society: all situations which are potentially likely to cause depression in anyone. Depression may also be caused by any of these situations.

- Physical causes such as:
    (i)   having recently had an operation
    (ii)   illness, especially viral infections
    (iii) head injuries
    (iv)   brain disorders such as a stroke or epilepsy
    (v)   hormonal fluctuations during and after the menopause
- Social causes such as:
    (i)   loneliness and isolation, e.g., the elderly living alone
    (ii)   lack of money resulting in loss of status
    (iii) bereavement
    (iv)   family changes, e.g., close family moving away

Depression takes on many forms and it is likely that the majority of cases are missed by the medical profession. Carers need to be aware of any changes in behaviour that may be a symptom of depression. Behavioural changes that may be symptomatic of a bout of depression include:

- feeling sad, upset and tearful; the patient looks sad and may frequently cry
- changes in sleep patterns causing the patient to get less sleep which, in time, makes them more depressed
- feelings of anxiety, often accompanied by sweating, heart palpitations and dizziness; anxieties

that may develop include a morbid fear that they have a serious illness (hypochondria), and feelings of guilt and/or persecution
- loss of appetite
- apathy about their everyday lives, a loss of interest in sexual matters and events going on around them, and an inability to concentrate or remember things
- loss of self-interest; they neglect themselves, and may not wash, dress or keep their homes clean
- plans to commit suicide
- mood swings where they may be very depressed and then change to being very 'high'; this is called hypomania.

Treatment for depression varies according to the needs of the patient and the views of the doctor (see Table 3.1). Here are some of the methods of treatment.

- *Counselling help* Individual or group psycho-therapy, where the patient's past and background are discussed to find out the possible cause of their depression, may be helpful to many depressed elderly people.
- *Drug treatment* Drugs may only be given on a doctor's prescription. Drugs used to treat depression (see Table 3.1) are very dangerous and it is important that they are taken as instructed and that only the person they are prescribed for takes them.
- *Electro-convulsive therapy* (ECT) Although ECT is generally frowned upon, it is sometimes used in serious cases of depression. The treatment is carefully monitored and the patient usually only suffers temporary side-effects such as headache

Table 3.1 Drug treatment for depression.

Group	Dosage	Comment	Possible side-effects
Tricyclic anti-depressants	Up to 2–3 weeks to take effect, start with low dose	Work by physically altering chemicals in the brain to prevent depression	Drowsiness, confusion, constipation, dry mouth, blurred vision
Monoamine oxidase inhibitors Anti-depressants		More powerful; less frequently used as more likely to have side-effects	Rise in blood pressure if taken with certain foods
Amphetamines		Alter mood without dealing with cause of depression	Likely to lead to dependence
Lithium	Given over a long period of time	Works by reducing mood swings; works on a long-term basis	

and possible loss of memory. Although these side-effects usually pass quickly, they can be quite severe. The patient is given a short acting anaesthetic and a muscle relaxant while an electric current is passed to the brain via the temples. The treatment is generally given twice a week for three weeks and is usually successful if the depression is a disease and not the result of circumstances such as bereavement.

Summary of keypoints

- The four major health problems faced by the elderly today are heart and circulatory diseases, cancer, arthritis and brain disease.
- Urinary incontinence should be medically investigated to find the cause. If the problem cannot be treated, continence management can help the patient cope with the problem.
- The likelihood of heart disease can be increased by genetic factors, an unhealthy diet, smoking, a stressful lifestyle and high blood pressure.
- Strokes, which can range from mild to severe, are caused by a blockage in the blood supply to the brain or a haemorrhage in the brain.
- The elderly are prone to respiratory disorders as there is usually a loss of resistance to infection.
- Digestive system diseases are frequently more difficult to diagnose in the elderly so any symptoms, however mild, should be reported to a doctor.
- Eyesight should be regularly checked in order to detect some of the more serious eye problems, i.e., glaucoma or blindness caused by diabetes.
- Teeth and dentures should be regularly checked to prevent discomfort.
- Changes in the skin should be investigated as they can be a symptom of underlying health problems which, if left untreated, can become more serious.
- There are many bone and joint diseases which may cause discomfort and lack of movement. Generally speaking, the earlier these problems are diagnosed, the better the chances are for treating the disease. Regular exercise helps to keep bones and joints healthy.

Assignments

1.   Incontinence is quite a common problem in the elderly. Look into this problem in your area by finding out about the following points.

- What your local health service offers the elderly person with an incontinence problem.
  (i)   Is there a specialist advisor?
  (ii) Is she/he attached to a hospital or health centre on a rota basis?
- The number of people seeking advice from the service and whether it satisfies an adequate percentage of the need.
- How patients find out about the service.
- What methods of continence management are promoted, i.e.,
  (i)   habit reinforcement
  (ii)   provision of continence aids and the methods of payment
  (iii) help for the patient
  (iv) advice and support for the carers
- Whether the advisory service deals with faecal incontinence and, if so, how?
- What methods of assessment are used.

2.   Research into attitudes towards incontinence to find out how people regard the problem. You may wish to include some of the following points:

- awareness of the symptoms and causes
- awareness of the help available locally
- attitudes towards patients

Here are some people you may wish to ask:

- a cross section of age groups
- people dealing with the elderly in their work
- relatives of the elderly

3.   On page 12 there is a list of the factors contributing to heart disease. Find out about each in more detail and the way they make us more susceptible to heart disease. Invite someone to talk to your group about these factors. Suggestions for speakers include a community dietician (contact local hospital) or a general practitioner. Further advice can be obtained from:

- your local Health Education Authority
- The Chest, Heart and Stroke Association, Tavistock House North, Tavistock Square, London, WC1H 9 JE

4.   Strokes frequently affect the elderly and range from being fairly mild to fatal. Find out more about strokes, include:

- the causes
- the symptoms
- the various effects on the mind and body
- the treatment available locally
- the aftercare and rehabilitation available locally

You may find the information from the following sources:

- Community Health Council
- Health Education Authority
- local general practitioner
- hospital – including the occupational therapist
- The Chest, Heart and Stroke Association (see p. 23 for address)
- local support groups
- stroke sufferers and their families

5.   Check that you understand the respiratory problems affecting the elderly and the dangers of the elderly developing pneumonia. If there are any questions, ask a nurse or doctor with special responsibility for the elderly to come and talk to your group.

6.   Although the elderly do suffer from digestive disorders, a healthy diet can help to reduce the likelihood of many of these disorders. Work out a healthy diet for the elderly and find out how digestive disorders are reduced by healthy eating.

7.   Find out more about the effects of eye disorders on the elderly and the provision in your area to help those with sight disorders. Research the causes, symptoms and treatment of:

- glaucoma
- cataracts
- blindness caused by diabetes
- other sight disorders

Find out about the services offered to help partially sighted and blind elderly people in your area. Some ideas include:

- sight testing
- library facilities, e.g., talking books, large print books, talking newspapers, etc.
- help in the home
- daycare
- aids and adaptations

8.   The idea of false teeth often causes amusement, yet people, including the wearers themselves, are often unaware of many facts. Ask a dentist to visit your group to talk about how he/she caters for the needs of the elderly requiring complete or partial sets of dentures. The following are some points you may wish to include in your questions:

- why dentures are needed
- any counselling the elderly person may be offered
- how the teeth are measured, made and fitted
- aftercare

- how dentures should be cared for
- any problems

9.   Ask either a doctor or nurse with special responsibility for the elderly to visit your group, or arrange a visit to a hospital or health centre in order to find out the more common health disorders in the elderly. Include some of the following:

- ulcerated legs
- varicose veins
- shingles
- arthritis
- osteoporosis
- intermittent claudication
- falls and drop attacks

10.   There is a great deal of misunderstanding over the mental health of the elderly. Many people think dementia is an integral part of the ageing process and few people are aware of the wide range of brain disorders that may affect the elderly. Find out more about the variety of brain disorders that affect the elderly. Information may be available from:

- the mental health section of your local hospital
- doctors and nurses with special responsibility for the elderly
- the local care of the elderly unit or residential home for the elderly, if they have provision for the mentally frail elderly

Some of the brain disorders you may wish to cover are:

- depression; its causes, symptoms and treatment
- dementia, i.e., confusion, Alzheimer's disease and multi-infarct disease; include in your research recent evidence suggesting that a high level of aluminium in the body may increase a person's chances of developing Alzheimer's disease
- hallucinations, delusions and obsessions
- personality changes
- self-neglect

Find out what provision there is locally for the elderly with brain disorders. You may wish to ask the following questions.

- How are the elderly assessed if they are diagnosed to be suffering from brain failure?
- How are they treated, i.e., home visits, out-patients, daycare, admitted to psychiatric unit, etc.?

- What are the methods of treatment, i.e., counselling, psychiatric counselling, drugs, electro-convulsive therapy (ECT) or a combination of these?

11. Recognising depression in the elderly is often difficult because so many of the symptoms can be caused by other health disorders. Find out about the various therapies available for treating depression, e.g., psychotherapy, group and individual counselling and so on in your area.

4

CARING FOR THE ELDERLY

Before discussing the provision of care for the elderly, it should be stressed that the majority of the elderly live an independent life in their own homes. It is the minority who live in residential homes or care of the elderly units (see Fig. 4.1).

The elderly represent a complete cross section of society and the aim of care should be to give them the help and support they need to maintain their independence and individualism for as long as possible.

Patterns of ageing

There are, however, changes in the ageing population which have implications on the type of care that needs to be provided.

- In 1900 fewer than 1 in 20 people were aged over 65; in 1989 over 1 in 7 people were aged over 65.
- In 1989 1 in 104 people were aged over 85; in the year 2001 it is expected that 1 in 65 people will be over 85.
- In 1989 60% of the elderly were women, and this figure increases amongst the old elderly.
- In 1989 65% of the disabled were elderly.
- Elderly people use hospitals twice as much as those under 65.
- Over half of all hospital beds are occupied by the elderly.

The implications of these changes are given below.

- More residential homes will be needed.
- Nursing care should be available in nursing homes for the elderly who do not need the complete hospital services; this would free many hospital beds for more needy cases.
- There should be an increase in hospital provision for the increasing number of old elderly.
- Social services will need to allocate more resources to deal with the needs of the elderly.
- Primary health care will also need to provide more resources.

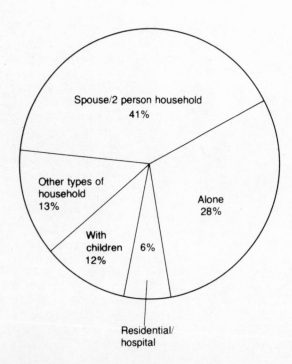

Fig. 4.1 Living accommodation in the elderly population.

What is community care?

Community care includes the help and support provided by the elderly person's family and the community and is a term frequently used when discussing the caring needs of the elderly. In the past, if there was no support provided by the family, the elderly were cared for in institutions. Recently there has been a move towards what is called 'community care', and this approach has also been adopted by those working with groups such as offenders, the mentally ill and the physically and mentally handicapped.

Community care was introduced for the following reasons.

- Living in institutions may lead to 'institutionalisation' and the the person may lose his/her independence and find it increasingly difficult to integrate into normal society.
- Medical advances now make it possible to treat certain physical and mental disorders so the elderly can remain at home.
- Moving the elderly back into the community saves local and central government money.

It is necessary to strike a balance between the ideal and the reality of community care. Ideally, the elderly person will be supported by friends and family, with back-up help from the Social Services and the Health Service. The reality, sadly, is not always this rosy. The Social Services and the Health Service are underfunded and understaffed and the responsibility of caring for the elderly either falls on the family (usually the woman), or the individual is left alone. At present, the general intention of government policy towards community care for the elderly is:

- to emphasise the role of the family
- to encourage private provision
- to encourage voluntary agencies by giving them funds redirected from the public sector agencies

The elderly in their own home

It is usually best for the elderly to stay in their own homes and be independent; this way they can keep their self-respect and dignity. But, in order to be independent, the elderly need reasonably good health, a suitable home and any social support that is necessary. The services responsible for providing this support are the Social Services Department and the District Health Authority. The Social Services Department is responsible for providing the following services:

- community care assistants (previously known as 'home helps')
- meals-on-wheels
- laundry services
- aids, adaptations and help for the handicapped
- daycare provision

- sheltered accommodation
- home care
- good neighbour schemes
- luncheon clubs
- night sitters
- welfare rights officers
- domiciliary occupational therapists

The District Health Authority is responsible for providing:

- primary health care teams
- hospital outpatients services
- care of the elderly hospital day centres
- shared care

These services are called 'domiciliary support services' as they aim to help elderly people stay in their own homes. Liaison and co-operation between the different carers is vital to ensure that the elderly receive plenty of support. The elderly clients' needs are assessed by a social worker who may recommend any one or more of the domiciliary support services.

The Social Services Department

Community care assistants

This is the most popular service and almost 90% of the clients are elderly. The role of the community care assistant is to clean, wash, shop and cook. The community care assistant organiser decides how many hours of help the client needs each week. Some local authorities make a charge for this service, depending on the client's means, whereas other local authorities provide the service free of charge. The community care assistant also provides a social role, giving the elderly client someone to talk to. Because the community care assistants know the clients, they are in a good position to report any mental or physical deterioration, so close liaison with a social worker is vital. Referrals for community care assistants come mainly from the Health Service, and social workers.

Meals-on-wheels

Meals-on-wheels are intended to give the elderly a well-balanced diet. The meals are distributed to the home or luncheon clubs, usually every other day, and they are frequently distributed by the Women's Royal Voluntary Service (WRVS), or other voluntary agencies. A small charge is made for the meals. Referrals for meals-on-wheels are made by the Health and Social Services.

STAFFS UNIVERSITY LIBRARY

Laundry services

These are provided to help district nurses, or relatives, cope with the large amount of washing needed if the elderly person is incontinent. Not all local authorities provide this service, and a small charge may be made.

Aids and adaptations for the disabled elderly

Aids such as walking frames, bathrails, non-slip mats, hoists, kitchen fitments, special cutlery, dressing aids and specially designed clothing are available (see p. 45–7).

Adaptations ranging from handrails and ramps to widening doors, chair lifts and a downstairs bathroom are provided with the local authority paying some or all of the cost. Occupational therapists assess the client's needs and make recommendations to the Social Services.

Daycare provision

Daycare is provided outside the elderly person's home. This may be in a residential home, a hospital or a daycare centre. The elderly person may attend daily, or less frequently, and transport is provided to and from the centre. At the daycare centre the elderly person will meet other people and take part in various activities, as well as getting a cooked meal at lunch time. The centre will also provide laundry services, hairdressing and chiropody (foot treatment) services. Therefore, the elderly living alone have some contact with the outside world, and those living with families will give the carer the opportunity to go to work or have a break. Referrals are made by the Health and Social Services.

Home care

This service may be provided by some local authorities to help the elderly who have come home from hospital and are particularly vulnerable. It includes a community care assistant, meals-on-wheels and home nursing for about four weeks after leaving hospital. After four weeks, the client is reassessed.

Good neighbour schemes

These schemes orginated in 1976 although, in practice, voluntary help for the elderly had existed for many years before that. They are run by voluntary agencies as well as the Social Services Department and aim to provide social contact, cooking, shopping, gardening and so on. The Social Services Department may make a small payment to the scheme.

Luncheon clubs

Luncheon clubs simply provide a cooked lunch three or four times a week for a small charge. These clubs may be held at community centres, church halls, day centres and so on, and help to get the elderly person out of his or her home to meet other people.

Night sitters

This service is provided by some local authorities to keep an eye on an 'at risk' elderly person during the night. The elderly person may be either waiting for admission to hospital or be seriously ill and the night sitter would be able to call a doctor or ambulance if necessary. Night sitters are often used to relieve the carer.

Welfare rights officers

The benefits system has always been complicated and, with the changes in the system introduced in April 1988, it has become increasingly complex. Some local authorities have a welfare rights officer who has up-to-date knowledge of the benefits and can offer help and advice to the elderly in need.

Domiciliary occupational therapists

Some local authorities provide occupational therapists who go into the elderly person's home and assess their need for aids and adaptations, although this service is not widely provided.

In general, the role of the Social Services Department is to co-ordinate the needs of the elderly client. The Social Services system varies from one local authority to the next and it is often a difficult task to make sure the client gets what help he/she is entitled to.

The District Health Authority

Primary health care team

Primary health care is the term for the medical staff

working in the community, usually in a general practitioner's practice or a health centre. The team, provided by the District Health Authority, consists of one or more of the following:

- general practitioner (GP)
- receptionist
- district nurse
- practice nurse
- health visitor
- midwife
- social worker (in some practices)

The elderly form a large proportion of the doctor's consultations and tend to need more home visits as they find it difficult to get to the surgery. District nurses are valuable as they can visit the elderly in their own homes and perform routine nursing tasks such as changing dressings, giving injections, medication and so on, while also keeping an eye on the patient's general condition. If necessary, the district nurse may then refer the patient for additional help, such as admission to a residential home or hospital, or recommend adaptations for the home or transport to a day centre. Because of these responsibilities, it is vital that the district nurse liaises closely with the Social Services Department.

The health visitor's role is to encourage the elderly person to remain healthy and independent by promoting good eating habits and offering help and advice when needed about all aspects of preventive health care. In addition to this, the other staff working closely with the primary health care team are dentists, opticians, chiropodists and occupational therapists.

More information on the primary health care team can be found on page 36.

Hospital outpatients service

If the elderly person develops a health problem, their GP may refer them to a specialist at a hospital, or arrange for them to have diagnostic tests. The elderly person may be offered help with transport to the hospital by volunteer drivers or by the ambulance service.

Care of the elderly units/day hospital

Care of the elderly units (no longer called geriatric units because of the poor image the term creates) offer the elderly person living at home the opportunity of coming to the unit for any number of days, or half-days, a week. They will be brought in and taken home by volunteer drivers or by ambulance, and at the care of the elderly unit they are offered nursing care, medical treatment, a meal, and a chance to meet other people. If the elderly person lives with relatives, it is also an advantage for the family as they will be relieved of some of the responsibility of caring for an elderly relative.

Shared or intermittent care

Shared care, although not generally available, is the term used for a care of the elderly ward which takes patients needing nursing care for 4–6 weeks, after which time the patients are returned home for 4–6 weeks. This happens on a regular basis and has many advantages:

- the patient does not become institutionalised
- the home carers are given a regular break
- two patients can use the same hospital bed

The voluntary sector

The fairly limited statutory provision given by the Health and Social Services needs to be backed up by voluntary sector provision. The voluntary sector includes friends and neighbours of the elderly person as well as voluntary and charity workers. Their role may be simply befriending and helping the elderly person and giving them contact with the outside world, or it may be organised on a local basis, for example community task forces doing gardening and decorating, etc. Charities and religious groups concerned with helping the elderly may build sheltered accommodation and day centres and offer other services such as holidays, hospitals, meals-on-wheels, the loan of medical equipment, mobile shops and libraries, and so on.

Community care, in all its forms, attempts to offer the elderly the opportunity of living an independent life within the community. There are, however, two major problems which are:

- the changing pattern of family life
- inadequate funding and staffing in the caring services

Recent times have seen the greatest proportion of elderly people living in their own homes. However, sooner or later the elderly people will need the support of the caring services which are, at present, underfunded and understaffed. With the move away from institutions, the burden of care will fall on the immediate family and this will cause major changes in family life over the next few decades.

When the elderly can no longer live independently

Many of the elderly live independent lives until their death, with perhaps some domiciliary support from the caring services and help from friends and relatives. A number will, however, need full-time care at some stage. This may be as a result of one or more of the following reasons:

- difficulty in continuing everyday life
- death of a partner
- a serious illness or operation
- onset of confusion
- coming home from a stay in hospital

This care may be offered by:

- relatives
- residential homes; either council or privately run
- care of the elderly units

Care in the home

Obviously there are many considerations to be taken into account before deciding to care for an elderly relative in the home, and these decisions should include the elderly person, as well as members of the family and professionals. The following points are some of the factors that may need to be considered.

- Who is to be the carer? Sometimes the answer is obvious, and sometimes it takes some discussion. Occasionally, the care may be shared on a rota basis, but the elderly person always needs to be consulted and needs time to decide.
- Is the carer able to cope physically and mentally with the added responsibility? If the carer has his/her own family, can the family cope with the increased demands of an elderly relative?
- How to accommodate the elderly person, whether in the carer's home, in an extension (a so-called 'granny' annexe), or whether a new property will need to be bought to suit the family.
- If the elderly relative is frail or disabled in any way, the home may have to be modified for them. Modifications may range from the simple to the more complex:
  - (i)   increased heating and lighting
  - (ii) access to bedroom, bathroom and toilet
  - (iii) modification to stairs, bath and toilet

Once the decision has been made there is still the need to constantly evaluate the situation. Is the elderly person being encouraged to remain as independent as possible? Are the members of the family happy? Is there plenty of outside contact for both the elderly person and the carer?

In many cases, the family manages to cope with problems and difficulties and, hopefully, makes use of the help available from the domiciliary support services (p. 27).

Sheltered accommodation

When it is no longer practical for the elderly person to live an independent life in their own home, sheltered accommodation may be provided by the Social Services Department. The accommodation is usually in self-contained flatlets linked to a warden by an alarm bell. The warden will call on the residents, usually twice a day, to check that they are all right. As the residents become increasingly frail, they may be transferred to a residential home for the elderly. Because sheltered accommodation is very popular, there is often a waiting list. The voluntary and private sector also provide sheltered accommodation housing schemes.

Residential care

For the elderly person being cared for by their family there may come a time when the family carer can no longer cope with the increasing amount of nursing involved, especially if the elderly relative becomes very frail or ill. There may also be other elderly people who do not have the opportunity of being cared for by relatives (either because they do not want to be dependent or because there is no suitable care available). In these cases, it is usually necessary for the person to go into a private council-run home or a voluntary sector residential home. Since the National Assistance Act 1948, local authorities have to provide full-time care for the elderly who cannot be cared for in the community, yet do not need hospital care. This is called Part 3 Accommodation. The elderly are admitted on a priority basis according to need and referrals are made by Health or Social Service workers.

Residential homes vary from area to area. Many are purpose-built to give the residents as much independence as possible, encouraging them to make their own drinks and snacks, etc, whereas others are run very much on the lines of an institution with fixed meal times, communal lounges and so on. Although some residents may return to their own homes or to relatives, the majority are there until they die or until they are admitted to a care of the elderly ward.

Because demand exceeds supply, many privately

run residential and nursing homes have been set up over the years. Private residential homes are vetted and registered by the Social Services Department of the district authority and private nursing homes are registered by the local health authority. Sometimes Social Services Departments have to send elderly people into private sector homes if there are no vacancies in the homes in their local authority.

The variety of residential and nursing homes is great but, in general, the residents tend to be frail and many will be confused. The attitude of the staff can make all the difference between the elderly person becoming either institutionalised and depressed, or feeling independent yet supported. The staff need to develop their own self-esteem through good working conditions, pleasant surroundings, in-service training and general respect. This helps to avoid the situation found in many residential homes where the elderly sit around idly staring out of the windows and are treated as if they were not in control of their faculties because of low staff morale.

Care of the elderly units

The majority of the elderly who need to be admitted to hospital (from their own home, the carer's home or from residential care) go to either a hospital specialising in care of the elderly, a care of the elderly unit or ward in a general hospital, a psychiatric hospital or to a specialist ward, i.e., an orthopaedic ward, to treat their particular disorder. Over the past couple of decades there has been a growing interest in the medical needs of the elderly and this is reflected by the general improvement in hospital care of the elderly. However, there are still a great number of problems which include the following:

- the general low status of nurses specialising in care of the elderly
- a high number of unqualified nursing staff
- too few specialists available, although the number has increased
- understaffing and underfunding
- bed blocking, i.e., the elderly have to remain in hospital, although they are technically well enough to be discharged, because there is nowhere for them to go.

The ideal care of the elderly unit should provide as many of the following services as possible:

- full-time nursing care
- daycare nursing
- physiotherapy
- occupational and rehabilitation therapy

- outpatients consultation
- investigative treatment
- leisure activities
- links with the outside world

About 60% of elderly hospital patients will go back into the community and the rest will either remain in full-time care or die as a result of illness or old age.

Although it is impossible to make generalisations, research has shown the following comparisons between private sector and council-run residential nursing homes to be generally applicable.

- The surroundings in hospitals and many local authority residential nursing homes tend to be quite institutionalised, whereas private nursing homes are usually more homely and provide more individual surroundings.
- Private nursing homes are more likely to offer single bedrooms, whereas only half of local authority homes, and virtually no hospitals, do.
- Most local authority and private nursing homes offer open visiting hours, whereas hospitals are frequently tied to the visiting hours applied to the rest of the hospital.
- Virtually all local authority nursing homes have a communal lounge, and the hospitals have a day room, whereas just under half the private nursing homes have no communal lounge facility.
- Patient choice over bedtimes, menus, making drinks and so on is limited in hospitals, a little better in local authority homes and generally good in private nursing homes.

There are, however, moves in many areas to improve the standard of care in council-run nursing homes by increasing the individual's privacy and improving decor, etc.

Summary of keypoints

- The majority of the elderly live in their own homes.
- The proportion of the elderly in the population is continuing to grow and this should mean a comparable growth in the support services.
- Nowadays there is a shift towards care in the community rather than in institutions. Sadly, the caring services in the public sector tend to be underfunded and understaffed.
- The elderly prefer to live independently for as long as possible and can be helped to do so by the support of the domiciliary services.
- Sheltered accommodation, provided by the

public, voluntary or private sectors, is a good balance of independence and privacy. At present, waiting lists for such accommodation are long.

- The provision of care by the voluntary sector plays a vital part in caring for the elderly. The services range from visiting and shopping to providing sheltered accommodation and residential homes.
- Caring for an elderly relative in the home demands a great deal of thought and planning which should include the elderly person as much as possible.
- The difference in standards of care in residential homes varies tremendously. It is a traumatic change for the elderly person to move to a home, and care needs to be taken to ensure that the move is made as smoothly as possible. People involved in arranging the transfer should ideally check that the home is, indeed, homely.
- Care of the elderly units have improved over the years and many try to make the patient's stay as pleasant as possible. Until recently, nursing the elderly was one of the least popular areas of nursing although much is being done to dispel the stigma that it holds.

Assignments

1. In the section 'Patterns of ageing' (p. 26), various statistics about the elderly have been given. Can you answer the following.

- Why are there more elderly people today than at the turn of the century?
- Why are there more elderly women than men?
- Why do the elderly account for more than half of the disabled population?
- Why are the elderly twice as likely to use hospital services?

2. With an increasingly elderly population, can you make suggestions that will help the community to provide adequate care.

- What resources should the primary health care team provide?
- What resources would the Social Services need to allocate to caring for the elderly?
- How should nursing homes be developed in order to free some hospital services?

3. What are the advantages and disadvantages of providing community care for the elderly rather than caring for them in institutions? Consider the

advantages and disadvantages from the point of view of the elderly person, their family, and society as a whole.

4. Provision for the elderly differs from area to area. In your own area, contact your Social Services Department and find out about local provision for the elderly. You may find that a social worker will be willing to come and talk to your group, or perhaps you will need to visit the Social Services Department. Make a list of questions you need to ask which may include the following.

- How is work with the elderly allocated, e.g., is there a social worker with responsibility for the elderly, or does every social worker have a generic training (i.e., covers all aspects of social work, rather than specialising)?
- What provision is there for the elderly in your area? For example:
  (i) meals-on-wheels
  (ii) community care assistants
  (iii) laundry services
  (iv) aids, adaptations and help for the handicapped
  (v) daycare
  (vi) residential homes
  (vii) home carer
  (viii) good neighbour schemes
  (ix) luncheon clubs
  (x) night sitters
  (xi) welfare rights officers
  (xii) domiciliary occupational therapists
  (xiii) other
- How do the elderly qualify for these services and are charges made?
- How are these services run, i.e., staffing, funding and so on?
- How are the elderly referred, i.e., by themselves, by the primary health care team, by neighbours, relatives, etc?
- Is there liaison between voluntary agencies, i.e., with individual social workers, meeting with Health Service personnel, etc?
- What are some of the ways that the service could be improved?

5. The Social Services Department is very complex and many elderly people do not receive the advice, help or financial benefits they are entitled to. How do you think the system could be altered to improve communication between voluntary agencies, the Health Service, the Social Services, the public and the elderly client?

6. Find out how the National Health Service (NHS) is organised in Great Britain. Include:

- the start of the NHS in 1948
- the reorganisation of the NHS in 1974 and proposed changes in 1989
- the roles of the Departments of Health and Social Security
- the services provided by the NHS
- Regional and District Health Authorities
- primary health care
- secondary health care
- Family Practitioner Committees
- Community Health Councils

7. Find out how the Social Services Departments are organised. Include the following:

- Local Authority Social Services Departments
- Probation Service
- Central government role (the Department of Health and the Department of Social Security)
- Local Social Services Departments
- Area Social Service Teams

8. Find out how the Health Service and Social Services Department liaise in your area.

9. What are the advantages and disadvantages of the following GP services for the elderly?

- a number of doctors in a group practice rather than one doctor running a local surgery
- an appointments system
- a receptionist

10. Look at the accommodation for the elderly in your area, for example:

- sheltered accommodation
- residential homes
- care of the elderly units and hospitals

Find out whether they are provided by:

- the council/public sector
- the private sector
- voluntary agencies (religious bodies, charities or organisations helping the handicapped)

(a) Arrange a visit to a residential home in order to find out more. Some questions you might like to consider are as follows.

- Is the home adapted or purpose-built?
- When was it built?
- How many residents are there?
- What is the average age of the male and female residents?

- Are there shopping facilities?
- Accommodation
  (i) Are the bedrooms single or shared?
  (ii) If shared, how many to a room?
  (iii) Are the bathrooms close by?
  (iv) Do residents have their own furniture?
  (v) Are there double rooms for married couples?
- Aids and adaptations
  (i) Is there a lift in the home?
  (ii) Is there any specially adapted equipment in the bathrooms to help the infirm to bath, shower or visit the toilet independently?
- Staffing
  (i) How many staff are there (day and night)?
  (ii) What are their duties?
  (iii) Are there part-time staff?
  (iv) Are voluntary helpers used?
  (v) Are there alarm-bells by the bed for night-time emergencies?
- Meal times
  (i) Are the meals provided or do residents have the opportunity to make their own drinks and meals?
  (ii) Are meal times flexible?
  (iii) Is there a choice of menu?
- Facilities
  (i) Are there facilities for hairdressing, dental treatment, sight testing and chiropody?
  (ii) Are these facilities free of charge?
- Can friends and relatives visit whenever they like?

(b) Arrange a visit to a local sheltered accommodation complex. Find out the following.

- When it was built
- Accommodation
  (i) Do the residents live in bed-sits or self-contained flats?
  (ii) Do they have individual or shared kitchens?
  (iii) Do they have individual or shared bedrooms?
  (iv) What is the role of the warden?

(c) Arrange a visit to a local care of the elderly unit. Find out the following.

- When it was built
- Whether it follows the same regulations as the rest of the hospital
- How visiting times are arranged
- The facilities the elderly patients are offered
- Recreational pursuits organised
- Whether it incorporates a day unit

STAFFS UNIVERSITY LIBRARY

- The number of patients in a ward
- Whether there is a day room available
- The role of the nursing staff
- Whether non-medical staff are employed

11.　Contact a local doctor's practice or health centre and ask if you can visit them or if one of the staff could come and talk to your group. Find out about the role of each member of staff that works with the elderly and also about the liaison with Social Services, dentists, opticians, chiropodists.

12.　The voluntary sector is separate from statutory agencies and profit-making agencies. Find out how the following voluntary agencies help the elderly in your area and add any other agencies you can think of.

- Women's Royal Voluntary Service
- Red Cross
- Help the Aged
- Age Concern
- Volunteer Agencies

13.　With the present emphasis on community, rather than institutional, care for the elderly, discuss in a group the short and long-term implications this will have on society, including both the family and the caring services.

14.　Having an elderly relative living with a family can have drawbacks for both the elderly person and the family. Consider these problems from the point of view of both parties and make a set of guidelines to help people cope in this situation. You may wish to consider the following points.

- The needs of the people involved, e.g., the elderly person, the carer, the carer's spouse and children.
- Financial arrangements, e.g., does the carer plan to continue to work? Does the home need any altering or adapting?
- The ability of the individuals concerned to adapt to the situation. Usually it is the child taking on the caring role and the elderly parent being cared for: a complex reversal of the parent and child situation.
- Can the elderly person cope with the upheaval?
- The ability of the carer to cope if the elderly person's condition degenerates, e.g., they may become incontinent, confused, and so on.
- The need to include the domiciliary services available.

15.　There is an emphasis today on the private sector in health care and this affects the provision of care for the elderly: sheltered accommodation and residential homes may be council or privately run. As a group, discuss the following statement: 'The best care is available if you have the money; if you don't there's only the state sector'. Is it right that state sector care should become a safety-net to those elderly people who do not have the money to pay for private care?

16.　Do you think the family has a duty to care for an elderly relative?

17.　Sometimes the carers dealing with the elderly (and this includes people from doctors and nurses to care assistants) tend to forget that the elderly have a right to be consulted about their everyday needs such as nursing, food, treatment, leisure activities and so on. The staff become task-orientated rather than person-orientated and emphasis is put on achieving tasks and making choices on behalf of the residents to create speed and efficiency at the cost of the elderly person's social and personal needs.

Write a job description for the ideal carer, including in your description some of the following areas:

- client involvement in the everyday running of the home or ward
- residents' choice (in menus, visiting, leisure activities, bedtimes, etc.)
- the need for client independence
- the role of the resident's family
- the role of the local community
- the need for efficiency versus the need to build-up personal relationships between staff and residents
- the need for routine

18.　Hospitals in some areas offer the following facilities to make caring for the elderly meet the needs of the elderly, rather than making the elderly take what is available.

- Day hospitals operate during the day only and offer medical treatment, nursing, chiropody, physiotherapy and occupational therapy, hairdressing and a cooked midday meal. Often patients can be treated and therefore do not need to be admitted to the full-time ward.
- Rehabilitation wards take patients who have been treated and may well go back into the community after physiotherapy, occupational therapy and/or general convalescence. Approximately half will return to the community, and the remainder will either go on to Part 3

Accommodation or die as a result of their illness.

- Slowstream rehabilitation wards offer a similar service to the rehabilitation wards but the patient is expected to make a slow recovery.
- Continuing care units are available for the patient who is unlikely to fully recover their physical or mental health. The patient has nursing care but is also encouraged to be involved in the community, where possible, by being taken out into the community or by people visiting the unit. Links with family and friends in the local community are encouraged.
- Five-day wards offer full-time nursing care, medical treatment and rehabilitation five days a week, and the elderly person returns home at the weekends.

Check which of these options your District Health Authority provides. Try and arrange a visit to each one and after your visit discuss the advantages and disadvantages of the facilities offered.

5

PEOPLE AND SERVICES CARING FOR THE ELDERLY

Caring for the elderly crosses boundaries and includes the Health Service and the Social Services as well as voluntary agencies, the family and friends. In this section the roles of the various people who come into contact with the elderly will be examined.

The Health Service

The Health Service is divided into primary and secondary health care teams. The primary health care team includes the people who the patient first consults about a health problem, and the secondary health care team usually includes the staff of the hospital where the patient is referred to when necessary.

Primary health care team

1. *General practitioner* A general practitioner (GP) is under contract with the local Family Practitioner Committee and a list of GPs can usually be found in post offices, libraries, Citizens Advice Bureaux, Community Health Councils and the Family Practitioner Committee offices. The list explains what services the doctor offers patients and how the particular surgery operates, i.e., surgery hours and so on. The role of the GP is both diagnostic and preventive:

- health checks
- prescriptions (certain drugs can only be obtained by prescription and the majority of the elderly are entitled to free prescriptions)
- referral to see a specialist, or admission to hospital
- recommending home visits to be made by the health visitor, district nurse, chiropodist, etc.
- diagnosing and treating health disorders
- advising patients about how to improve their physical and mental health

2. *District nurse* About half the case load of the district nurse are elderly patients. They are given nursing attention in their own homes so they can maintain independence for as long as possible. This nursing includes changing dressings, giving injections, giving bed baths, checking blood pressure, etc. The nurse will also visit at weekends if necessary.

3. *Health visitor* Although much of a health visitor's time is spent visiting mothers and young children, they do work with the elderly. Their role is to advise the patient and refer them on to other services that they may need, e.g., meals-on-wheels, voluntary organisations, etc. They will also be aware if the patient's health deteriorates.

4. *Chiropodist* The elderly are eligible for free chiropody (women over 60 and men over 65). The chiropodist treats various foot problems such as corns, bunions, and ingrowing toenails as well as recommending appliances and footwear.

Secondary health care team

Unless they are taken seriously ill or have an accident, the elderly will attend hospital as an outpatient or as an emergency admission.

As an outpatient, a GP will refer a patient to see:

- a specialist doctor, usually called a consultant, who specialises in certain parts of the body
- an outpatients' department for an X-ray, blood test, etc.

The results of the consultation or tests are sent to the GP who will then inform the patient.

As an emergency admission the patient will either be collected by ambulance, or admitted to hospital the same day following a telephone call made by the GP.

The following is a list of the many different types of hospital in Great Britain which may have facilities to cater for the needs of the elderly patient.

- Cottage hospitals which are small and usually have a limited range of facilities.
- Psychiatric hospitals which cater for the mentally ill and usually have a large number of elderly patients.
- Mental handicap hospitals.
- Day hospitals (see p. 29).
- District general hospitals which have many wards and services, including a care of the elderly ward. Many of the elderly will, however, be treated in specific wards such as orthopaedic, surgical, medical and so on.
- Hospices are hospitals especially for the terminally ill and dying and are often run by voluntary or religious organisations to cater for the physical, mental and spiritual needs of the dying patient and their family.
- Private health care includes clinics, hospitals, GPs, nurses, alternative medicine, health screening check-ups, dental treatment, eye tests, nursing, chiropody, prescriptions, consultants, psychiatric treatment and care of the elderly. In other words, the same services as the NHS offers are available, but the patient has to pay for it. The patient can pay by putting money into a private health scheme, usually British United Provident Scheme (BUPA) or Private Patients Plan (PPP), over a number of years. By paying for treatment as it is needed, the elderly tend to use the following private medicine provision.
  (i) Private nursing where the nurse is in the elderly person's home and cares for them on a full-time or part-time basis.
  (ii) Private hospital treatment is used to avoid the sometimes lengthy waiting lists that the NHS hospitals have. Many elderly people go into private nursing homes which may offer medical care, surgery, and care for the mentally ill old person. If there is only nursing care available in the private nursing home, the patient's own GP will visit them if necessary.

As private medicine involves either payment into a scheme, or enough money to pay for treatment, it is only available to a minority of the elderly population: the vast majority use the NHS services.

Details of the staff found in the average general hospital

1. *Doctors* Usually there are specialist doctors, consultants, who run a team of doctors which includes the following.

- Consultants are responsible for all the treatment (drugs and/or surgery) the patient receives in hospital. He/she visits the patient in the ward to check on their progress.
- Senior registrars deputise for the consultant.
- Registrars carry out operations.
- Senior House officers carry out operations under supervision and prescribe drugs.
- House officers are new doctors who intend to work in a hospital or become a GP. House officers are the doctors who have most to do with the patients and they may also prescribe drugs.

2. *Nurses* who may be either enrolled nurses (EN) or registered general nurses (RGN). Nurses may also specialise in caring for the elderly.

3. *Physiotherapists* use exercises and activities in order to:

- treat diseases affecting the bones, joints and muscles
- help prevent disorders worsening
- treat injuries, such as broken bones, to help the patient return to normal
- help keep the patient mobile

4. *Occupational therapists* use activities to help treat both physical and mental illnesses in order to encourage independence. They may help stroke patients, the disabled and handicapped, and people affected by muscle, joint and bone diseases.

5. *Psychologists* find out how people react and adapt to various situations. The elderly may use the services of a psychotherapist who treats diseases through the patient's mind using any of the following methods:

- suggestion, i.e., the patient has an idea suggested to him/her by the psychotherapist
- persuasion, i.e., appeals are made to the patient's reason
- analysis, i.e., half-conscious or subconscious memories are brought to mind
- group therapy, i.e., patients are treated as a group using argument, discussion and drama
- education and employment

6. *Psychiatrists* are doctors who specialise in treating mental illnesses.

7. *Speech therapists* help treat speech disorders caused by accident or illness. In the elderly, speech is often impaired by a stroke.

8. *Hospital social workers* (previously called

almoners) offer practical help and advice to those ready to leave hospital. The help and advice covers aspects of financial support, domiciliary services, and aids and adaptations that are available for the home.

9.　*Anaesthetists* are doctors who specialise in the field of anaesthetics. The elderly mainly come in contact with the anaesthetist before and after any surgery requiring a local or general anaesthetic.

10.　*Radiographers* take X-rays and computerised scans to detect illness or injury.

11.　*Medical laboratory officers* are the people who check samples of blood, urine, sputum, stools, etc., from slides and swabs to detect illnesses.

12.　*Dieticians* work out special diets needed by particular patients in hospital and will advise the patient how to cater for their dietary needs once they have been discharged. Special diets may be needed by the obese, diabetics and people suffering from diseases of the kidney.

13.　Other staff, such as auxiliary nurses and porters, help with the everyday running of the hospital.

The Social Services

The Social Services are funded by the Department of Health (DoH) and the Department of Social Security (DSS). The social worker is likely to have many elderly people in his/her case load, and their intention is to help the elderly person maintain his/her independence for as long as possible in the following ways:

- social activities to prevent feelings of loneliness and isolation; the social worker will co-ordinate local activities provided by the Social Services, the NHS and voluntary agencies (p. 29).
- visits to day centres or day hospitals (p. 28).
- the provision of aids and adaptations in the home
- financial advice on the benefits available
- meals-on-wheels (p. 27)
- admission to a residential home if necessary
- the provision of other domiciliary services (p. 27–9)

Voluntary agencies

These vary from area to area. There are national agencies which have a special interest in the elderly such as Age Concern, Help the Aged, and other societies dealing with special needs, e.g., the Alzheimer's Disease Society and the Chest, Heart and Stroke Association. All these are able to offer help and advice to the elderly and their families. They also have local provision that may help the elderly such as a volunteer bureau, or a local branch of a charity.

Information can be obtained from various sources and the following are some examples.

- Charities Digest
- Directory of Associations } Found in the local library
- Voluntary organisations

- Social Services
- Community Health Council
- Citizens Advice Bureau } Address and telephone number found in local telephone directory
- Volunteer Centre
- Health Education Authority

Family and friends

Family and friends caring for the elderly person need help and support in practical, emotional and financial matters. Apart from the statutory help provided by the NHS and Social Services, they may also find help and support from people in the same position as themselves. Further information on support groups can be obtained by contacting the National Council for Carers and their Elderly Dependants.

Other agencies

1.　*Dentist* The elderly need to visit the dentist twice a year, and more frequently if there are problems. Even if they wear dentures, these should be checked about once a year. Most dental treatment is free of charge for the elderly.

2.　*Optician* Eyesight deteriorates with age, so the elderly need regular eyetests both to check their eyesight and detect whether their eyesight is being affected by diseases such as glaucoma (p. 16), diabetes (p. 16) or high blood pressure (p. 12).

3.　*Pharmacist* The local pharmacist can offer advice to the elderly as well as dispensing prescriptions for medicines and appliances.

Summary of keypoints

- Caring for the elderly crosses all boundaries: interdepartmental between the Social Services and the Health Service; inter-agency, including voluntary and statutory agencies, and family and friends. The needs of the client should be paramount.

- The Health Service is divided into primary and secondary health care teams. The members of the primary health care team are those people first consulted by the patient, and the secondary health care team is made up of the staff of the hospital that the patient may be referred to.
- The Social Services, although liaising with the Health Service, has the aim of helping the elderly maintain their independence for as long as possible by offering financial advice and organising domiciliary support.
- Voluntary agencies offer help to the elderly and often fill gaps left by the statutory services provision.
- Family and friends will usually do most of the caring and need practical, emotional and financial help and support.

Assignments

1. Find out about provision for the elderly in your area.
- What services does the GP or health centre provide?

- Arrange a visit to the health centre to find out about the everyday work of the health visitor and district nurse.
- Find out what hospital provision there is, i.e.:
  (i) day hospital
  (ii) general hospital
  (iii) psychiatric hospital
  (iv) hospice
  (v) private clinics, hospitals or nursing homes
  (vi) care of the elderly unit

2. Find out the various specialisms a consultant can practice in.

3. Contact the Social Services Department to arrange to talk to a social worker about local provision for caring for the elderly.

4. Visit your local volunteer bureau, or Citizens Advice Bureau to find out what voluntary provision there is for the elderly and their families.

5. Contact a local pharmacist and ask him or her to explain their job and how they may be able to help the elderly.

6

DEATH AND BEREAVEMENT

Being with someone who is dying is a demanding experience, mentally, emotionally and physically, and very difficult to imagine unless you have been through it. In many cases, the death of an elderly person is the result of a long illness and at other times the death may be sudden and unexpected. However much the death is planned for, it is never easy to adjust to or come to terms with.

The death of a person touches many people: the carer(s), the family and friends, and the dying person themselves. It is not possible to generalise about death and its effects, but there are some factors that are common to people facing the situation, and these will be looked at later. It is usually better if the person dies in the familiar surroundings of their own home with their close family near at hand. If this is not possible and the person dies in hospital, nurses are trained to care for the needs of the dying patient and to deal with the close family.

The role of the carer

The carer needs to help the patient die with dignity and comfort. Obviously this includes physical, mental and emotional or spiritual needs. The patient needs to be free from pain and suffering and in a comforting and sympathetic environment. In many cases the patient's medical and nursing needs are taken care of by the doctors and nurses, and the mental and emotional needs are met by the close family with support from medical staff.

As a society, we are fairly unfamiliar with death and the topic is usually swept under the carpet in an attempt to pretend it does not happen. Talk of death is considered to be morbid and people who have been bereaved are often avoided because of embarrassment. Because we do not talk about death, we tend to regard it with fear. Meeting people who are dying makes us aware of our own mortality, so we may try to avoid contact with them. The carer needs to think about their own attitude towards death as they need to be a support to the dying patient. If a carer finds working with the dying difficult, they need to talk to a professional about the problem.

The dying person

The majority of the elderly die peacefully, having come to terms with the idea of death and possibly even welcoming it at the end of a long illness. There is often an opportunity to say goodbye to their families which is very satisfying and supportive to the relatives. Others may be less lucky, and the carers (who may be the family) need all the help and support they can get if the death takes many weeks to come.

Towards the end of an elderly patient's life, the doctor may decide to no longer treat their illness because the treatment is doing more harm than good. This decision is made in conjunction with the family, close friends, nursing staff, and the patient themself, if this is possible. However, to make the patient as comfortable as possible, treatment for symptoms and pain will continue. The person caring for the terminally ill patient needs to be aware of some of the medical and nursing treatment available.

1. *Pain* Almost all pain can be treated nowadays, so there is no need for the dying patient to be frightened of pain. Pain caused by problems such as pressure sores, indigestion, etc., can be cured by treating the symptoms. The pain of terminal illness can be helped by giving regular doses of pain-killing drugs. The drowsiness caused by these drugs usually wears off after a few days.

2. *Stomach disorders* Some diseases may cause sickness which can be treated by giving an anti-emetic (anti-vomiting) drug. The carer should make sure that the patient is as comfortable as possible during and after bouts of sickness.

Diarrhoea and constipation can also be treated. Constipation is better treated by diet, otherwise it can be relieved with the use of mild laxatives, suppositories or enemas if necessary.

3. *Shortness of breath* Drugs can be given to help breathless patients breathe, but the carer will need to help the patient to find a comfortable position by arranging pillows and backrests. The patient may even need to sleep sitting up in a chair in order to get as much breath as possible.

4. *Difficulty in swallowing* This problem is frightening for the patient and the carer and occurs when the muscular walls of the oesophagus gradually cease working. The patient will need to be fed very liquid foods, or food drinks.

5. *Everyday nursing care* Nursing the dying patient needs particular care. Every action should be explained and the patient's wishes listened to. The nursing is the same as for any bed bound patient and includes:

- washing
- changing clothing
- continence management
- mouth care
- moving to avoid pressure sores
- giving food and drink
- shaving
- emotional support

Emotional support is vital as the dying patient may need to speak frankly at times about his/her fears, feelings and questions. Many dying people develop a need for some sort of religious support as they approach death, even if they have not been religious in their earlier life. This support can be found in the ministers of the various Christian denominations, and all hospitals have a chaplain who will visit the sick and dying. Moslems, Jews, Hindus and other faiths will all have their own religious representatives who will help comfort the dying of their faith. The carer and the close family can be very supportive just by being there and holding the patient's hand and listening to anything they have to say.

Coping with death

When a patient realises he/she is going to die, they go through certain recognised stages.

1. A refusal to recognise that they will die. This denial may take the form of disbelieving the doctor's diagnosis, anger, or the idea that they are dreaming.
2. Anger when they wonder why they have been singled out for suffering.

3. Bargaining, i.e., promising to live a good life if they are allowed to live a little longer.
4. Depression as the truth gradually sinks in. When this happens the patient may become anti-social and cry a great deal. They are not necessarily depressed just for themselves, but also on behalf of the people they are leaving behind.
5. Acceptance when the patient has come to terms with approaching death and reaches a sense of peace.

The death

As death approaches the patient becomes weaker and no longer wants to eat or drink. They are usually unable to move and lose their reflexes, so the carer will need to check for pressure sores and for signs of incontinence. As the blood circulation slows, the extremities become mottled and blueish and the skin, although cold to the touch, sweats profusely as the body temperature rises. The patient will be hot, although they feel cold to the touch.

As the senses fail, the window curtains should be left open to allow more light to get in and people around should talk clearly. It is reassuring to hold the patient's hand. Sometimes a patient may lose consciousness, while others may be conscious to the end. Breathing tends to become erratic (this is called Cheyne-Stokes respiration) and the rate of respiration slows down and sometimes stops for up to half a minute before starting again. Cheyne-Stokes respiration may last for days. At this stage, the close family will have been called to the bedside, and their needs should be considered too. The family need regular breaks for food, drinks and rest as the strain is very demanding. At the moment of death, the patient stops breathing and becomes limp.

It is then the home nurse or carer's job to:

- close the patient's eyelids
- note the time of death
- contact the GP
- replace any dressings with clean ones
- cover the patient with a sheet
- contact the undertaker

If the patient has died in hospital, the body will be taken to the mortuary.

The bereaved

Losing someone close is a very traumatic experience and the bereaved go through various stages of grief before they can come to terms with the death. Immediately after the death, the relatives may want to be left alone with the patient for a while. It has been found that if the bereaved person is able to grieve properly, then he/she will be better able to accept the death, and be less likely to become mentally or physically ill. So 'putting on a brave face' and bottling up feelings of grief is likely to have a detrimental effect on the bereaved person.

As with the dying person, the bereaved have similar phases that they need to go through in order to come to terms with the death.

1.   A refusal to believe the person has died. Questions are asked like, 'How can she be dead, I only saw her an hour ago?' This stage of shock and denial may last from a few days to weeks.
2.   Anger and resentment that they have been left alone to cope; a feeling of 'How could you let me down like this?'. Alternatively, there may be anger about the fact that the dead person has died when it should have been someone else.
3.   Bargaining, as the bereaved person weighs up what it would be worth to have the deceased person back again.
4.   A period of deep depression may follow, usually together with loss of appetite, weight loss, sleeplessness and a lack of interest in life. This is when the bereaved person needs plenty of help and support from family and friends. It is not unusual for physical illness to develop at this stage as resistance is low.
5.   Acceptance of the death and an ability to remember what the dead person did in life rather than concentrating on the death.

If grief is not permitted for one reason or another, various problems can arise so people around the bereaved person need to be sympathetic to their needs. The bereaved can be helped by bearing in mind the following guidelines.

- To come to terms with death, the bereaved need to believe the person is dead. Seeing and touching the dead person can be helpful, and the funeral or cremation is a symbol that death really has occurred.
- Try to avoid the use of drugs to help the bereaved cope with grief. Drugs, including prescribed drugs, alcohol and cigarettes, may give temporary relief but the cause of the sadness is still there and needs to be coped with.
- Be willing to ask for help, advice and support. Practical help immediately after a death can be obtained from the undertaker, and help with financial details from a solicitor, Citizens Advice Bureau or the agencies dealing with the bereaved. The DSS publish a leaflet called *What to do after a death*, and there are books and booklets published by *Which?* and other agencies. CRUSE, The National Organisation for the Widowed and their Children offers practical and emotional support and advice to bereaved families.
- The bereaved will be in particular need of support at times like Christmas, the deceased's birthday and anniversaries, etc.

Practical arrangements after the death

1.   *Registering the death*   All deaths have to be registered and there must be a doctor's certificate which gives the cause of death. If the doctor has not seen the dead person before their death, the coroner will need to be informed and he/she will decide whether to issue a death certificate or recommend a post-mortem examination. If the death occurred in suspicious circumstances, the coroner may decide to carry out an inquest which will decide the cause of death. Once the relative has the death certificate, he/she can go to the local registrar to register the death. The death must be registered within five days of the death in the registration sub-district that the death took place in. The person going to the registrar's office, called the informant, is usually the relative who was there at the death, or one who lives in the locality of the registrar. The informant needs to answer various questions including:

- names, surname(s) and sex of the deceased
- time and place of death
- the deceased's address
- the deceased's full-time occupation and whether retired
- the deceased's medical care

When the details have been checked they will be entered into the register of deaths, signed by the informant and countersigned by the registrar. The death certificate is needed to make certain claims. The certificate is a copy of the register entry and can be obtained from the registrar for a small fee.

2.   *The coroner*   The coroner is either a doctor or a lawyer or occasionally both and his/her main role is to investigate any deaths that have been reported to him/her. Deaths among the elderly may be reported to the coroner for any of the following reasons:

- if the doctor has not visited the person for 14 days before the death (28 days in Northern Ireland)

- if the death is caused by industrial disease or war injury
- if the death was sudden and unexplained
- if death occurred in suspicious circumstances
- if death may have been caused by
  (i) neglect
  (ii) any type of poisoning
  (iii) any abuse
- if death was caused by suicide
- if death occurred during an operation or before coming to after an anaesthetic

The coroner will arrange for a post-mortem to be carried out and then, if still unsatisfied, an inquest. The majority of elderly people's deaths do not need the services of the coroner.

3. *The funeral* The decision whether to be buried or cremated is usually made by the deceased before they die. If not, the next of kin needs to decide.

Undertakers, usually called funeral directors, organise the complete funeral or cremation. The undertaker collects the body from the home or mortuary, and will lay out the body if it has not already been done by the nursing staff.

- *Laying out the body* This should be done as soon as possible after death. The body is washed, and shaved if necessary, and the orifices are blocked with cotton-wool. The dead person is dressed in clean clothes, the eyelids closed and the jaw supported to prevent it sagging. The undertaker may well embalm the body as this delays the onset of decomposition. The blood is replaced by chemicals which temporarily preserve the body and help it to look peaceful. The undertaker will ask the relatives what to dress the deceased in, either their own clothes or a shroud, and will take the body to the chapel of rest.

The funeral either starts from the deceased's home or the undertaker's premises, depending on where the body is, and the body is taken to the cemetery or crematorium. After the service the body is either cremated or buried.

After the funeral there will be tasks such as settling the will, claiming life insurance and pensions and transferring ownership of property and other possessions, all of which entail contacting various agencies at a time when the bereaved are still in a state of shock. Useful names and addresses offering help and support are given at the end of the Assignments section (see p. 44).

4. *Suicide* In old age the suicide rates for men and women alter. In younger life, more women than men commit suicide, yet the number gradually alters at middle age. With men, the number of suicides continues to grow into old age. This is thought to be because men are less able to adapt to the loneliness and isolation of old age. In very old age there are few suicides as people seem to accept the limitations of their bodies. Coping with a suicide is particularly hard on the bereaved who have had no time to adjust to the death, so they will need a great deal of help and support.

5. *Euthanasia* Euthanasia, or mercy killing, is a very controversial issue. People see it as two extremes; the enforced killing of all elderly or infirm people, or the right to die with dignity when you wish.

In Holland, many doctors practise euthanasia. Terminally ill patients with no hope of recovery make a decision, along with their family, that they would like to die. The doctor then administers a drug that will kill them. Although technically against the law in Holland, doctors are rarely prosecuted as they are considered to have acted in the patient's best interests.

In Great Britain, euthanasia is still against the law and doctors will not actively 'kill' a patient. They will, however, withhold certain treatment that may cause the patient pain and discomfort at the end of a terminal illness if it is in the best interests of the patient. A pressure group who believe in euthanasia, EXIT (Voluntary Euthanasia Society), offer help and advice to terminally ill patients and their families but, in general, the majority of the population are against euthanasia on the grounds that it would be abused.

Grief in other societies

Western society has made death into a taboo subject in recent years. In the past when death was more frequent and usually took place in the home, it was a part of everyday life. Today, as most people die in hospital, death and grief have become more embarrassing because people do not know what to say. There is no longer any ritual associated with death which could give us a pattern to follow. Other societies handle death, grief and mourning in very different ways according to their religious beliefs.

Summary of keypoints

- Death and bereavement need to be dealt with

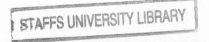
STAFFS UNIVERSITY LIBRARY

with care and tact. All those involved (the carer, family, friends, and the dying person) need counselling, help and support.
- Much of the pain and discomfort associated with terminal illness can be alleviated by medication.
- The carer needs counselling so that they are able to deal with the patient's emotional needs.

Assignments

1. Discuss the role of the carer when dealing with the dying person. The carer may be a member of the family, the spouse, or a professional nurse. Discuss the needs of the dying person and their family

2. Find out about care of the dying in your area by arranging to talk to one or more of the following people:
- a member of staff in a hospice
- a hospital chaplain, or a minister of any denomination
- a person who has lost someone close (be tactful about your approach)
- a district nurse
- a bereavement counsellor working for a voluntary agency

3. The stages of grief outlined in this chapter; denial, anger, bargaining, depression and acceptance can be applied to all cases of loss. Discuss these feelings. Why do you think they are fairly universal?

4. Find out how other religious communities cope with the death, grief and the disposal of the body of a relative or friend, for example:
- Islamic
- Hindu
- Buddhist
- Jewish

5. Contact a local funeral director and ask whether he/she would be able to come and talk to your group about their work.

Useful names and addresses of agencies offering help and support to the bereaved:
- Age Concern England, Bernard Sunley House, 60 Pitcairn Road, Mitcham, Surrey CR4 3LL (01–640 5431)
- CRUSE The National Organisation for the Widowed and their Children, Cruse House, 126 Sheen Road, Richmond, Surrey TW9 1UR (01–940 4818/9047)
- Hospice Information Centre (BHC), St Christopher's Hospice, 51 Lawrie Park Road, London SE26 6ZZ (01–788 1240)
- National Council for Voluntary Organisations, 26 Bedford Square, London WC1B 3HN (01–636 4066)

Some books on death and bereavement:
- Copperman, H. (1983). *Dying at Home*. John Wiley & Sons, Chichester
- Kubler-Ross, E. (1973). *On Death and Dying*. Tavistock Publications, London
- Lamerton, R. (1980). *Care of the Dying*. Penguin, Harmondsworth
- Speck, P. (1978). *Loss and Grief in Medicine*. Bailliere Tindall, London
- Which Publications. (1986). *What to Do When Someone Dies*. Hodder & Stoughton, Kent
- Worden, J.W. (1983). *Grief Counselling and Grief Therapy*. Tavistock Publications, London

6. Discuss the use of euthanasia for the elderly, terminally ill patient. Do you think there is a place for euthanasia in this country?

Find out about euthanasia in Holland and the work of EXIT in this country.

EQUIPMENT AND ADAPTIONS FOR THE DISABLED ELDERLY

The use of equipment and adaptations can help the disabled elderly person live an independent life in his/her own home so that they only need help and support from family, friends and the domiciliary services. This idea is also in keeping with the recent move away from institutionalised care. Although equipment and adaptations can be bought by the individual, some may be supplied to the elderly by the Social Services and the Health Service. There is a vast range of equipment and adaptations available from a simple set of cutlery to complete kitchens, stair lifts, gardening equipment and outdoor transport. The disabled elderly person really needs to try out any equipment he/she may want to buy as there is a wide choice. If possible, they should visit one of the disabled living centres around the country to try the equipment out. Much of the equipment is zero-rated for value added tax (VAT) which means that no VAT will be charged, for example:

- medical and surgical appliances
- adjustable beds
- chair and stair lifts
- adapted motor vehicles
- commodes and other toilet equipment

Further details can be found in the *Directory for Disabled People*, published by Woodhead-Faulkner in association with the Royal Association for Disability and Rehabilitation. The directory also gives plenty of information about choosing equipment, claiming back VAT, employment, leisure interests, holidays, education and so on.

Equipment and adaptations encourage independence in all areas of life. The following are some of the more common aids available.

1. *Personal hygiene*

- Rubber safety mats can be used in the bath and shower to prevent slipping.
- A sloping bathrail is more secure and allows the

person to gradually lower themselves into the bath.
- A bathseat or bench allows the person to swing themselves into the bath and sit on the seat whilst washing. This makes it easier for the person to get out of the bath afterwards (see Fig. 7.1(a) and Fig. 7.1(b)).

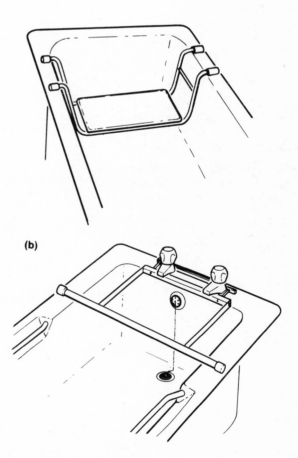

(a)

(b)

Fig. 7.1 **(a)** Bath seat. **(b)** Bath rail.

- A toilet rail situated beside the toilet helps the person to lower themselves on to the toilet (see Fig. 7.2).
- A raised toilet seat helps the person to get up from the toilet (see Fig. 7.3).
- Washing aids such as a long-handled sponge, a tap turner, nail brush with suction pads, a flannel mit with a pouch for soap, and a long-handled toothbrush are a few of the ideas that help to make washing easier.

2.   *Dressing and undressing*   There are many simple ideas that can help make the task of dressing and undressing easier, e.g., using Velcro instead of fasteners such as zips and buttons on bras, shirts, ties, cuffs and so on. Front opening clothes should be chosen as these are easier to do up and loops should be attached to socks and tights to make them easier to pull up.

3.   *In the kitchen*   There are aids available for cooking and eating. People who have a poor grip, perhaps caused by arthritis, need thicker handles to hold, whereas people with the use of one arm only need a plate surround to push against whilst eating. Other aids include teapot stands for easy pouring, spiked breadboards for holding a loaf of bread steady whilst slicing, non-slip mats and suction pads, one-handed trays, saucepan guards on cookers, clip-on aprons, jar openers, etc. (see Fig. 7.4).

4.   *Mobility*   Moving around the house may pose problems and mobility aids range from a simple walking stick to a stair lift.

- Walking sticks should be the correct height with the handle at hip level. Some walking sticks have a tripod on the bottom for greater stability and they are also suitable for those learning to walk again after an injury or operation.
- A walking frame gives more support than a stick.
- Ramps fitted over steps are easier for wheelchair access.
- Extra rails help when fitted at strategic places, i.e., by the front door, on the stairs, by the telephone and so on.

5.   *Leisure*   The elderly disabled still need leisure interests. There are aids available to make hobbies like gardening possible, and pencils and pens can be made easier to hold by putting a thick elastic band around them for gripping. Various voluntary agencies for specific disabilities will be able to offer help and advice about coping with everyday life, and the addresses can be found in the *Directory for Disabled People* (see p. 48).

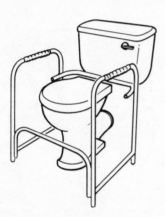

Fig. 7.2   Rails around a toilet.

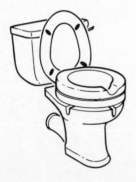

Fig. 7.3   Raised toilet seat.

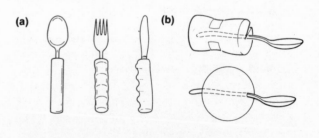

Fig. 7.4   Eating aids (a) Manufactured eating aids. (b) Improvised eating aids.

6. *Outdoor mobility* There are various schemes available locally and nationally that aim to help the disabled get out and about for which many of the elderly disabled are eligible.

- *Help with public transport fares* Many local authorities give concessionary fares on local buses; they may be either free or at a reduced price. Further information can be found at the local town hall or by contacting a social worker. The local authority will also offer help if a person has to attend hospital for treatment, and information about this can be found at the local DSS office.

  British Rail is usually able to accommodate people in wheelchairs, but there are no disabled toilets on trains; mainline stations do, however, provide disabled toilets. There are some concessionary rail fares available.

- *Help with wheelchairs* Wheelchairs can be borrowed from various voluntary agencies, such as the British Red Cross Society, but they are usually borrowed from the Disablement Services Authority, which is under the District Health Authority. However, Social Services do loan out wheelchairs if necessary. Wheelchairs will be loaned and maintained for the disabled elderly if the person's doctor recommends its use. In certain cases an electric wheelchair will be supplied.

- *Buying a car* It is unlikely that many elderly disabled people will want to buy a car, but there are many schemes available to help the disabled buy their own car. One example is the Mobility Scheme, a charitable organisation that helps the disabled lease a car using their mobility allowance.

  The Orange Badge Scheme allows the disabled to park more easily by relaxing certain rules and regulations. They can park for an unlimited time at meters and restricted parking areas and may have free parking at certain places of interest. The Orange Badge Scheme disc (see Fig. 7.5) is supplied by the local Social Services Department. Many car dealers will give discounts to disabled drivers, so it is worth contacting the local Social Services head office to find out which car dealers offer this service.

- *Mobility allowance* This benefit is a non-contributory and non-taxable cash benefit that is paid every four weeks to people unable, or almost unable, to walk because of physical disability. Information on this allowance can be found in a local DSS office.

- *Safety in the home* Although vital to everyone, safety in the home has a particular importance to

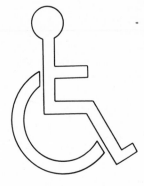

Fig. 7.5 The orange badge scheme symbol.

the elderly disabled as they are more likely to have an accident in the home. Common sense precautions can help prevent the likelihood of accident and injury. For example:

  (i) not putting mats on polished floors
  (ii) making sure carpet corners are held down
  (iii) keeping stairs well lit
  (iv) using a fire guard
  (v) checking that clothes are flameproof
  (vi) using a kettle with an automatic cut out switch
  (vii) keeping the temperature indoors warm and wearing enough clothes in winter
  (viii) wearing non-slip footwear

With the support of family, friends, and the domiciliary services to keep a check on safety and to suggest aids and other means of making everyday tasks easier, the elderly disabled person can be encouraged to be independent for as long as possible.

Summary of keypoints

- Equipment and adaptations can help the elderly person to remain as independent as possible.
- The equipment may be bought by the individual or supplied by the National Health Service, Social Services or voluntary agencies.
- Care should be taken when choosing equipment and comfort and safety should be major considerations.

Assignments

1. Arrange a visit to the Disabled Living Foundation, 380 Harrow Road, London W9 21N (01-289

6111) or one of the centres around the country (addresses in the *Directory for Disabled People*). Telephone beforehand to check that they have a wide selection of equipment and adaptations available and that the centre can accommodate your group.

2.   Find out whether your local Social Services Department or the Health Service offers the loan of equipment and adaptations to the elderly disabled.

3.   There are many books available outlining the type and availability of equipment and adaptations. The Oxfordshire Health Authority, for example, publishes detailed books on equipment for the disabled (contact Equipment for the Disabled, Mary Marlborough Lodge, Nuffield Orthopaedic Centre, Headington, Oxford OX3 7LD (0865 750103)). Look at some of the books that are available to find out about the wide range of equipment that is produced.

4.   The list of ideas for making the home safe for the disabled elderly person (p. 46–7) is by no means complete. Devise a set of home safety guidelines to cover all parts of the house and garden.

5.   Find out the concessionary fares available to the elderly handicapped person in your area. You may need to contact the Social Services Department or the local bus station.

6.   Contact British Rail to find out how they cater for the disabled elderly traveller.

7.   Find out more about the Mobility Scheme and how it operates. Are there any elderly disabled drivers who have taken advantage of this scheme in your area?

8.   Visit your local DSS to collect information on the mobility allowance.

   Useful addresses:

*   Royal Association for Disability and Rehabilitation (RADAR), 25 Mortimer Street, London W1N 8AB (01-637 5400); co-ordinates voluntary organisations helping the disabled and offers information on mobility
*   Motability, 2nd Floor, Gate House, West Gate, The High, Harlow, Essex CM20 1HR (0279 635666)

9.   As a group discuss the specific problems the elderly disabled may encounter. Much of the information on equipment and adaptations available for the disabled is geared towards the younger disabled person; the elderly disabled have the added problem of old age. What special considerations do you think they need in terms of:

*   personal hygiene
*   dressing and undressing
*   the kitchen
*   mobility
*   leisure
*   safety in the home
*   outdoor mobility

8

A HEALTHY OLD AGE

One of the aims of this book is to help people to understand that ageing does not necessarily go hand in hand with physical and mental deterioration and loss of independence. The vast majority of elderly people live independent and fulfilled lives and they have the same needs and interests as the rest of society. As people become more elderly it is obvious that they are likely to have some health problems, but in most cases these can be treated and, hopefully, not affect the person's quality of life too much.

Diet

Healthy eating applies to everyone from the newborn baby to the very old. The old myth that the elderly should be offered a light diet of steamed fish and milk puddings has, hopefully, been dispelled. Unless they have some digestive disorder that is affected by what they eat, the elderly can eat a normal diet. Over the years, however, the idea of what constitutes a 'good' diet has changed. After the Second World War people were encouraged to eat refined foods and plenty of meat for protein. In the light of more recent research, we are now advised to eat a diet high in unrefined foods and to get our protein from pulses and low fat meat and fish. This may be a problem for some elderly people who believe that the post-war type of diet is better for them. Help and advice from a doctor, community dietician and the media may persuade them to change, but in some cases the elderly person may prefer their usual diet.

The greatest dietary problem facing the elderly is poor nutrition. The elderly population most at risk are those who are over 70 and housebound, the old elderly (80 +) and widowers. The elderly living with a family or in residential care tend to have a better standard of nutrition. Poor nutrition is caused by one or more of the following factors.

- Loss of appetite, which may be caused by:
  (i) mental disorders, e.g., confusion, dementia and/or psychiatric problems

  (ii) physical disorders that make preparing and cooking food impractical and difficult, e.g., arthritis, blindness or partial sight, an inability to move and being housebound
  (iii) social problems, e.g., feelings of loneliness, bereavement and apathy
  (iv) the after-effects of illness, particularly viral infections
- Lack of money to buy food which may be caused by a genuine lack of money, when priority may be given to paying for heating, etc., or because the elderly person has not budgeted well.
- Certain drugs which affect the appetite in one of two ways:
  (i) the person feels nauseous so does not want to eat
  (ii) the drug affects the body's ability to absorb certain vitamins and minerals so vital nutrients from food are not absorbed
- Lack of knowledge about what is needed in a healthy diet.
- Drinking too much alcohol which affects the way the body absorbs vitamins.
- Taking laxatives; this is a habit that some elderly people may have started many years ago when it was thought that you were constipated if your bowels were not opened at the same time every morning.

Poor nutrition is dangerous in the elderly as it gives them a low resistance to illness and a reduced ability to cope with any problems. If they do become ill or injured, or if they are not eating a balanced diet, their health is more likely to decline after treatment than improve. It is not always easy to recognise that an elderly person is inadequately nourished, and the problem may go on for years. The following are some of the disorders caused by poor nutrition.

Constipation

This term has always caused disagreement. Constipation really has nothing to do with the frequency of bowel movement. Some people open their bowels three times a day, whilst others do so only once every three days; each is normal for the individual concerned. Constipation is actually the hardening of stools because of a delay in reaching the rectum. The causes of constipation are:

- lack of fibre in the diet
- lack of fluids
- lack of exercise
- regular use of laxatives
- not opening the bowels when you want to and 'holding on'
- taking certain drugs

In the elderly, constipation can lead to faecal impaction (see p. 15) so it is important that the problem is dealt with as soon as possible. The following are some guidelines to help prevent constipation.

- As much exercise as possible should be taken, with the general health and fitness of the person also taken into account. Advice on exercise can be found at local community education offices, the Health Education Authority, doctors' surgeries and so on.
- Plenty of liquid should be drunk. Many elderly people cut down on the number of drinks they have so they do not have to visit the toilet so often. Incontinence sufferers cut down in the vain hope that it will cure the problem. However, the elderly should be encouraged to drink 1–1½ litres (2–3 pints) of liquid a day.
- Laxatives should not be used unless they are prescribed by a doctor.
- A diet high in fibre should be eaten. Some suggestions are:
  (i)   high fibre bread
  (ii) skins left on vegetables where possible
  (iii) wholemeal flour used in baking instead of bleached white flour
  (iv) plenty of fruit and vegetables
  (v)   high fibre breakfast cereals where possible

Anaemia

This condition is found when the blood becomes low in haemoglobin, the material that gives blood its red colour and which carries oxygen in the blood. The symptoms of anaemia are:

- tiredness
- shortness of breath
- pale skin
- heart palpitations
- sleeping disturbances
- dizziness
- loss of appetite
- headaches and disturbed vision
- swelling of the ankles
- chest pains

The two most common types of anaemia found in the elderly are:

- iron deficiency anaemia
- pernicious anaemia

Iron deficiency anaemia, which is the most common, is usually caused by internal bleeding from, for example, haemorrhoids, or stomach ulceration caused by certain drugs. The internal bleeding means that iron is lost and is not absorbed into the bloodstream. It is treated by increasing the iron-giving foods in the diet and iron tablets are given. If the anaemia is very severe, a blood transfusion may be necessary.

Pernicious anaemia is caused by poor absorption of vitamin B_{12} in the diet because the stomach does not produce the substance (intrinsic factor) needed to aid the absorption of vitamin B_{12} from the food eaten. The disease is treated by having a vitamin B_{12} injection every month.

Vitamin C deficiency

A severe form of vitamin C deficiency (scurvy) is rare nowadays, yet the elderly may suffer from a lack of vitamin C in their diets. Those who have a vitamin C deficiency are more likely to bruise easily and wounds take longer to heal. Vitamin C is found in fresh fruit and vegetables, and the causes of deficiency are:

- eating institutionalised foods, e.g., meals-on-wheels, hospital or residential home meals; these meals tend to be overcooked, and this kills the vitamin C content
- not going out to buy fresh fruit and vegetables
- lack of knowledge about the importance of vitamin C in the diet

The following are some guidelines to ensure that the elderly person gets enough vitamin C in their diet:

- eat an orange or grapefruit each day, or drink fresh fruit juice
- drink blackcurrant juice with added vitamin C

- eat fresh potatoes, or instant mashed potato with added vitamin C, as these are high in vitamin C
- eat foods containing vitamin C everyday (elderly people are less able to store vitamin C in their bodies for long periods)

Vitamin D deficiency

Vitamin D is found in sunlight, in milk and in liver. Our bodies store the vitamin D gained from the summer sunlight to last us through the winter. Vitamin D is needed to transport calcium from the food we eat to our bones and a lack of vitamin D will cause a type of rickets called osteomalacia. Vitamin D is needed in old age as the bones tend to become more brittle as a natural part of ageing. The elderly are likely to suffer from vitamin D deficiency because:

- they may be less likely to go out, especially if they are housebound, and therefore miss the opportunity to absorb the sunlight
- they may wear a lot of clothes because they feel the cold, leaving no part of their body exposed to the sunlight
- they may not eat food high in vitamin D

Guidelines to help prevent vitamin D deficiency are:

- eat foods that are high in vitamin D, such as oily fish, milk, liver, eggs and malted drinks
- make sure the elderly get plenty of fresh air and are not too well covered

A well-balanced diet should, hopefully, eliminate most of the dangers of poor nutrition. What the elderly person needs from their everyday foods is all the essential proteins, carbohydrates, fats, vitamins, minerals and fibres, but in adequate quantities; too few will lead to being underweight and too many will lead to obesity. It is also important to remember that, as people get older, fewer calories are needed to maintain the same weight.

Sometimes the elderly will have special dietary needs, either as a result of illness or surgery, so they will need help to prepare a diet plan that is easy to follow and fits in, as far as possible, with their everyday lives:

- diabetics need to have a carbohydrate and fat controlled diet to create a stable blood sugar level
- renal failure sufferers need to limit the amount of

protein they eat in order to put less pressure on the kidneys
- people suffering from high blood pressure or heart disorders need to eat a low fat, low salt and low sugar diet

Exercise

Exercise is vital in old age and it has many benefits including:

- a lowering of blood pressure
- increase in muscle strength, including the heart and lungs which are muscles
- increased efficiency of the lungs
- an improvement in co-ordination and balance
- a reduction in stiffening of the joints
- a reduction in the build-up of cholesterol likely to clog up the veins and arteries
- psychological benefits, including a lower incidence of depression and a general feeling of well-being
- a reduction in the level of certain diseases which are exacerbated by lack of exercise, e.g., obesity, brittle bones, diabetes, arthritis and other joint diseases, certain circulatory diseases, high blood pressure and lung disease

At no stage in life should a big exercise programme be started if a person has always been fairly immobile, and the elderly are no exception. Exercise needs to be started gradually, depending on the person's physical health at the start and a doctor's advice should always be listened to. A person suffering from arthritis is going to need to perform different exercises from a thoroughly healthy young elderly person, and the doctor or physiotherapist will advise them on what to do. The recommended exercises are swimming, walking, keep fit and so on, and many Health Education Authorities run exercise classes for the elderly. The following are some guidelines for exercising.

- Before starting anything new in the way of exercise advice should be sought. People suffering from certain health problems may already be doing exercise routines as part of their therapy.
- Exercise classes may be offered by the local Community Education Department, often in conjunction with the Health Education Authority and District Health Authority. Some sports and recreation centres offer classes for elderly people, and the advantages of classes aimed at the older

STAFFS UNIVERSITY LIBRARY

person is that the exercises are geared towards their needs. The elderly are recommended to follow these guidelines before exercising:

   (i)   always take care to warm-up properly before exercising

   (ii) do not eat for at least 1 ½ hours beforehand

  (iii) do not exercise if feeling unwell or very tired

Pastimes and interests

Everyone needs one or more interests that help them to relax and take their mind off everyday matters. The elderly are no different in this way and they also benefit from the relaxation, stimulation and, often, the social side of having interests both inside and outside the home. Clearly, age and health greatly affect the type of hobbies and interests the elderly can follow, yet people tend to be well aware of their limitations and choose something that is possible to do and does not cause them frustration.

The following factors need to be considered when choosing a hobby or interest.

1. *Health* Strenuous activities are unlikely to interest an elderly person suffering from arthritis, and an elderly person with poor eyesight is unlikely to want to do an activity that demands close work. Unfortunately, deteriorating health may force some people to change interests that they have had for many years, but they may find something better suited to their present situation. Usually, however, people are able to decide what best suits their physical capabilities.

2. *Finance* Some leisure interests cost a great deal of money, whereas others are virtually free. Finances need to be considered to prevent stressful problems.

3. *Reasons for taking up leisure interests* People take up interests for various reasons. Some decide to exercise to improve their health and fitness, others take up an interest purely to meet other people, whereas some choose pastimes that demand thought, skill and/or expertise in a particular field. It is important that the elderly person decides what is required from an interest before they get involved in something that may not fulfil this need.

4. *Time available* Some leisure interests can be done at any time and anywhere, whereas others, perhaps because they involve other people, have a set time and place. Sometimes keeping a commitment like this is not always possible and will need to be considered.

Finance and budgeting

The elderly are, on average, more likely to be on the poverty line than most other members of society. The elderly today all receive the minimum state pension, and many have private pensions that they have taken out when working. However, with today's rising costs, their income often falls short of their needs. People working today are more likely to be better off financially when they retire as many pensions are index-linked (they increase in line with the rate of inflation). There are many problems caused by a lack of money: poverty is a vicious circle that affects all aspects of a person's life, and the elderly are usually less able to cope with the stresses poverty causes. The following are just some of the ways that poverty can affect the elderly.

- Elderly people are less likely to have certain basic requirements in their homes, e.g., fridge, washing machine, bathroom, central heating and so on. Clearly, this is not due only to lack of money (they may never have had these amenities when they were younger) yet in old age they are less able to cope without these things. A lack of these basic amenities means the elderly person is more likely to neglect him/herself and become undernourished and unhealthy.
- The home is less likely to be safe and maintenance gets neglected.
- Less money may be spent on food, leading to poor nourishment (see p. 49).
- Heating may be switched off to save money, with the high risk of hypothermia and other health problems associated with a cold environment. Research has shown that hypothermia is associated with poverty and inadequate housing.
- People who are poor feel inferior to the rest of society and the elderly are no different in this respect. They may feel particularly bad if they have become increasingly poor and need to accept financial help from the DSS or their family. They will tend to feel a loss of independence, and socially embarrassed in front of other people.
- Mentally, poverty can cause great stress and the elderly are not able to cope with high levels of stress. Over a length of time, stress can cause mental and physical illnesses.

In the past, the State did not help the elderly and the poor elderly were usually faced with having to go into the workhouse if they had no family to care for them. Workhouses were established as a result of the 1834 Poor Law Amendment Act which was introduced in order to deal with unemployment. This Act worked on the principle of 'less eligibility', i.e., the conditions in the workhouses should be worse than the worst conditions found amongst the poor. Workhouses, therefore, acted like a punishment for being poor and separated the sexes, even if married, and gave people tedious work to do and fed them unpalatable food. The idea of pensions was not introduced until 1908 when a small, non-contributory pension was given to the needy over 70, depending on the results of a means test. Contributory pensions were first introduced in 1925 and, over the years, the system changed greatly which made it very complex and difficult to administer. Because of the wide variety of pension schemes available and the diversity of the present Income Support system, more detailed work on pensions and benefits is in the Assignment section at the end of the chapter (see p. 62).

Income Support was introduced in April 1988 to replace Supplementary Benefit. The introduction of the new system caused a great deal of controversy: media coverage suggested many people would be worse off and others would lose their benefits altogether and, in many cases, this seems to be the case. Further research in the Assignment section (see p. 62) will help each person to find out the situation in their area.

A background to Income Support.

- The law behind Income Support is the Social Security Act, 1986. Details about the Act and regulations are made by the Secretary of State and approved by Parliament. Copies of the Act may be found in local libraries, or bought from Her Majesty's Stationery Office or bookshops.
- The regulations are often updated and amended and these details are available in various leaflets which give information on the financial support available. These leaflets can be found in GPs' surgeries, Social Services Departments, Citizens Advice Bureaux, walk-in centres, hospitals and so on.
- There is an Income Support Manual which deals in detail about how the system works. It can be found in public libraries, local DSS offices and advice agencies.
- If the client feels that they have not been dealt with fairly, an appeal can be made to the Social Security Commissioners.
- There are a series of Transitional Rules which were introduced to help people cope with the changeover from Supplementary Benefit to Income Support. These rules only apply to people who were claiming Supplementary Benefit before April 1988.

In general, people receiving Income Support have to be available for work. It is obvious that this and other regulations cannot be applied to the elderly, so the following is a brief outline of how the system is applied to the elderly.

- People over 60 do not have to sign on for work.
- Income Support is affected if the person is living in a Social Services funded residential care or nursing home, or is in hospital for any length of time. The DSS no longer pay the person Income Support but pay the cost of the residential care or nursing home and give the person some money for everyday spending.
- Premiums (special additional payments) may be made for pensioners aged between 60–79.
- Higher pensioner premiums may be made for people aged 80 and over, and to those of 60 and over if either member of a couple is receiving one of the following:
  (i)   Attendance Allowance
  (ii) Mobility Allowance
  (iii) Invalidity Benefit
  (iv) Severe Disablement Allowance
  (v)   Registered Blind Allowance
  (vi) Provided with a disabled person's vehicle
- Housing benefit may be paid to those people responsible for housing costs. Methods of payment vary depending whether the home is privately owned or rented from a council or private landlord.
- Assessment of Income Support depends on the person's income (the weekly amount coming in from work, benefits, maintenance and so on) and capital (savings, investments, lump sum payments and the value of the land and property owned, but not lived in, by the person). Disregards is the term used for any income which is completely or partially ignored in the assessment.
- Benefits which are ignored when assessing Income Support are:
  (i)   Housing Benefit*
  (ii)   Attendance Allowance
  (iii) Mobility Allowance
  (iv)   Christmas Bonus
  (v)   Constant Attendance Allowance
  (vi)   War Pensioners' Mobility Supplement
  (viii) Exceptionally Severe Disablement Allowance

(vii)   Severe Disablement Occupational Allowance

(ix)   Social fund payments

*   This is only ignored if it is not paid in respect of residential care or nursing home fees.

- The first £5 of total income from the following benefits is ignored:
  (i)   War Widow's or Widower's Pension
  (ii)   War Disablement Pension
- Certain special incomes are ignored:
  (i)   gifts of up to £250 in a 52 week period
  (ii)   annuities from, for example, the Victoria Cross and George Cross
- People receiving Income Support are entitled to:
  (i)   free dental treatment
  (ii)   money off vouchers for glasses
  (iii)   free prescriptions
  (iv)   help with the cost of travelling to hospital

The system is a very complex one and, although there are many leaflets about each benefit available, the elderly person would be best advised to seek advice from either their local Department of Social Security office, Citizens Advice Bureau, social worker or charity dealing with the elderly.

Retirement

It is very easy to see retirement as being the end of a useful working life and the beginning of loss of independence. Compulsory retirement, which operates in this country (usually 60 for women and 65 for men), is a time of stress for many people. It is often seen as:

- losing friends and colleagues from work
- needing to live on a reduced income
- a loss of status in a society that tends to value people in terms of the work they do
- becoming part of 'the elderly' and receiving various benefits and concessions

All this comes at a time when many older people are coming to terms with other life situations such as:

- less than perfect health
- family moving away
- death of friends and family

It is important that people are prepared for retirement and all that it brings in terms of mental, physical and social changes. Many areas run pre-retirement classes as part of their community education provision, and the forces and some private companies run courses to prepare their employees for when they stop work. However, the majority of today's elderly people have already retired and have had little or no help to prepare them for what to expect. Insight into what they feel would benefit all people dealing with and caring for the elderly, both on a professional and a family basis. Research has found that for many people work gives them an aim in life and offers an outlet for motivation and ambition, as well as fulfilling a social and economic role. Without it people tend to feel useless, and this applies to both the unemployed and the retired. However, there are people who look forward to retirement, and make plans to retire as early as possible from the work scene, and it is to be hoped that this positive approach towards retirement will increase in tomorrow's elderly population.

The following are some guidelines to help people cope with the prospect of retirement. For people already retired, many of the suggestions are still valuable. Retirement should be planned for in the following areas:

- finance
- courses
- leisure interests
- health matters
- where to live/housing
- social needs

Personal relationships

Society seems to give very little consideration to the personal relationships of the elderly: they are assumed to have no problems as they are not seen to have the same needs in relationships as younger members of society. The majority of books about the elderly fail to even mention relationships, and this only reinforces the idea that the needs of the elderly are mainly to do with caring for the body rather than the emotions. There are a number of variables to bear in mind when considering the personal relationships of the elderly because of the widely differing needs of a 65-year-old and a 90-year-old person:

- some people will be married couples who have grown older together
- some will be alone through death of a partner, divorce, or through never having married
- some will have a physical or mental disorder

At present, the majority of the elderly are either married, or widowed because of bereavement. However, in the future this pattern will change because of the more recent trends of increasing divorce rates and less pressure on people to marry.

Relationships are to do with loving, and growing older does not affect the way we express our feelings. Affectionate people remain affectionate and the less demonstrative stay that way; what does alter is our attitude towards relationships.

When people are younger, a relationship tends to have different priorities. In adolescence, the sex drive is very strong and physical attraction plays an important role in a relationship. In all societies, most couples then go on to get married and have a family. Couples tend to have a family when they are in their 20s as they are best able to cope with the physical and mental demands of parenthood. As the family grows older, the children leave home and the parents have to cope with many changes, including a loss of their children's dependence on them, their own ageing, and a change in emphasis in their own relationship. Compatible couples are happy to have more time to spend together without so many family demands. Their relationship will tend to become more firmly based on companionship and shared interests as they will be by now completely comfortable in each other's company. Less happy couples may find the extra time they have to spend together too demanding, so they may plan their lives independently of each other. Unmarried people, and couples with no family, are unlikely to be confronted with these major changes in role.

Sexually, there are certain physiological changes brought about by ageing, but these need not affect a person's attitude to their sexuality. What is more likely to do this is the general attitude of society that the elderly have no sex life and all they need out of a relationship is companionship. This need not necessarily be so, and it is up to the individual concerned to make up his or her mind about their approach to sexuality. The following are the most common physiological changes in sexuality caused by the ageing process:

- women reach the menopause during middle age (usually around 45–50 years) and their menstrual cycles gradually stop as the ovaries stop producing eggs
- men continue to produce sperm, but there are fewer healthy sperm, and less volume of semen
- a man's erection takes longer to develop, is less firm, and not so frequent as in youth
- women may have a drier vagina as the lubricating process slows down
- orgasms for men and women are less powerful
- men and women take longer to become sexually aroused

- there may be a loss of libido (interest in sex) in both men and women

These physiological changes are not necessarily problems and couples can easily adapt to them as they do, after all, come on gradually. Couples who carry on an active sex life into old age (and there are many of them) are less likely to have any problems as regular use of the sexual organs is the best way of keeping them in good working order. The other advantages of maintaining an active sex life are that the individual feels more desirable, which increases self-confidence, and has a feeling of fulfilment and satisfaction and sex is a very enjoyable activity for a couple who find pleasure in each other's company. Indeed, many elderly people find that their sex lives have improved and suggest the following reasons:

- no fear of pregnancy
- no need to 'prove' yourself
- increased self-confidence
- more time available
- no family around making other demands

Family relationships

Not all the elderly have family to consider, but the majority do and, even if they do not have children of their own, they generally have brothers and sisters with families. There is no doubt that the role of the family has changed considerably in the West over the past few years. The following are some of the changes that have occurred over the past decades.

- Fewer children being born, probably because of improved birth control and women's desire to work.
- The number of nuclear families has increased. In the past, and in less-developed countries today, the extended family made many demands on women as they had to care for the children, the sick and the elderly.
- Women's position in society has changed. Women no longer need to rely on men for financial support, so they are not obliged to get married.
- Families are more mobile than in the past because of the need to find work and because of improved transport. It is no longer unusual to find families separated by hundreds of miles.
- The role of the State has changed. The Welfare State provides much that was undertaken by the

family in the past, including caring for the elderly.

These changes affect the present-day elderly who may well have childhood memories of how the elderly were cared for by the family. However, research has shown that the vast majority of today's families offer a great deal of help and support to elderly relatives, although this is not always without its problems.

Growing old has its difficulties for the ageing parent and the child. The parent is used to being the one with wisdom and experience and the child may have often turned to him/her for advice, help and support. The child is used to looking up to the parent, and often relying on them in times of need. With ageing, however, comes a change in role. Often the elderly parent needs the help and support of the child, and the child needs to come to terms with the idea that they can no longer rely on the parent. This may create resentment on both sides as it is a difficult situation to accept. The ageing mother loses her role as confidante and the ageing father may lose his role as 'head of the household', all of which cause stress and tension. An awareness of these problems on the part of the ageing parent and the child should help to prevent the problems from becoming unmanageable.

Grandparenting is another area that can be a benefit to the family or a cause of much stress and anguish. There are many complex relationships going on in even the most straightforward family set-up; a daughter or son-in-law, a daughter-in-law and son, the other grandparents, and so on. There are also additional potential problems if the family have been through a divorce and remarriage where there may be additional children, second wives or husbands, etc. Not all people are reasonable and tolerant, so perhaps honesty when discussing the role of the grandparents is the best way of preventing trouble spots.

Friendship and loneliness

Socialising is a fundamental necessity in order to keep an interest in life. People who do not mix socially are likely to become introverted, depressed and lose interest in everyday life and their appearance. The problem with much of the social provision for the elderly is that it is associated with stereotyped images such as 'Darby and Joan' clubs and day trips to the sea. Many elderly people themselves have been heard to say, 'I can't go there, everybody is so old'! A wide range of social activities is probably the best way

to broaden people's horizons. The elderly are, however, increasingly likely to have to cope with various problems. Many of them, mainly women, are coping with the loss of a partner and there is an increasing likelihood of infirmity for both sexes. Both these situations are likely to hinder them going out and meeting other people, so they may increasingly withdraw from society.

Loneliness, which is a very negative and destructive emotion, may develop as a result of this isolation and, if left to grow worse, can lead to mental and physical illnesses. Loneliness can be coped with by the younger, more healthy elderly person who may be able to come to terms with the fact and realise that they do need to get out and about. The older elderly, especially those who are infirm, will have greater problems because they will need to rely on other people to alleviate their loneliness.

In many ways, it is a good idea to psychologically prepare ourselves as early as possible for the time when we may be alone. Developing interests that are our own and can be continued in some form into old age can help to mentally prepare us for the time when we may have only our own company for much of the time. Suicide rates have shown that women are better able to cope with loneliness in old age than men. This is probably because in our society women have looked after the home and family and are able to look after themselves. The older men, however, are more likely to have been cared for by women throughout their lives and are less able to cope with caring for themselves after their wives have died. They will also have had to come to terms with retirement, whereas many women in today's elderly generation are unlikely to have worked for any length of time and can, therefore, cope with the additional leisure time more easily.

Guidelines to help prevent loneliness and isolation are as varied as the situations elderly people live in. The independent elderly couple, the widow or widower in good health, the ageing parent living with his/her family, the elderly person living in a residential home, or a care of the elderly unit: all these people have widely differing needs and interests so no rules can be made to prevent them feeling lonely. Those who come into contact with these people, either on a professional, social or family basis, need to remember that they are individuals who have a right to make their own decisions. This should not be used as an excuse for leaving them alone, but it should be considered when planning anything social for the elderly. They can be persuaded, encouraged and motivated, but not forced.

Generally, the following ideas may give some insight into the problems faced by the elderly.

- Loss of hearing and sight leads to a great sense of isolation. The deaf person cannot hear people talk easily, either directly or via the television, radio, music, theatre, cinema and so on. The blind or partially sighted person cannot enjoy television, cinema, theatre, handicrafts, mobility, getting dressed and so on. People with speech problems also suffer because other people find it difficult to understand them.
- Sensory problems, as explained above, isolate the person because other people tend to avoid communicating with them as it takes more effort and causes many people embarrassment.
- Sight, smell, taste, touch and hearing can be stimulated by friends and family. Bright colours, strong smells, tasty food, etc., can all help to make the elderly person more aware of their surroundings and less likely to feel cut-off and isolated.
- Pets are a good idea if the person is physically able to care for them. The responsibility of caring for an animal has been shown to be beneficial to the elderly as they feel needed and loved.
- A wide variety of company is best, from children to people of their own age, as mixing mainly with people of their own age can lead to insularity (a decreasing awareness of the rest of society).
- Loneliness does not mean being alone. It is possible to be lonely in a crowd, whereas you can be alone and quite content.
- The elderly can become isolated by geography, e.g., living in the country with no transport, living far away from friends and family, living in fear in the city, etc.
- Bereavement can cause emotional isolation.

Housing

Housing is one of the areas where the elderly tend to be deprived. As the majority of the elderly live in their own homes, this can have far-reaching effects on their physical and mental well-being. The provision of good housing is a political issue and poses many moral questions such as whether everyone has a right to a certain level of housing, how it should be financed, what amenities are needed and so on. It is commonsense to be aware of the fact that the housing needs of the elderly are different in the following respects.

- The elderly spend longer in the home so the home needs to be safe and comfortable.
- They are more likely to suffer from minor or major health problems so the home needs to be warm, safe and clean.
- They need easy access to various public amenities such as transport, shops, doctor, library, etc.
- They may not have an adequate income to pay for repairs, maintenance and the everyday costs of running a home.
- The more suitable the home, the longer the elderly person can live an independent life. Various surveys have found that the elderly owner-occupier is more likely to need home repairs costing thousands of pounds and, as almost half owner-occupiers are widows living on pensions, these costs make the prospect of repair impossible. The elderly are also more likely to live in homes without basic amenities (i.e., indoor toilet, bathroom, etc.) and are often unable to pay for adequate heating. The elderly are the least able to cope with housing problems, especially if coupled with health and emotional problems, so help and support is needed from society to make any transition from their own home to a different residence easier to accept.
- Housing needs change with time. The elderly person needs to decide whether to adapt where they live or move somewhere more suitable for their changing needs.
- The prospect of limited mobility in the future needs to be considered.
- Everyday household items should be easily accessible and easy to use.
- Baths and toilets must be accessible.
- Moving home is very upsetting to most elderly people so it is often better to install aids and adaptations in their present home.
- Many elderly people keep their homes underheated in winter which adds to the risk of developing hypothermia. The elderly may not be aware of the cold as their sense of touch deteriorates (see p. 6) so a temperature reading should be taken at regular intervals.

It is important to be aware of the housing needs of the elderly. Independence is vital: housework, gardening, shopping and taking care of oneself is very therapeutic and beneficial. If independence is removed too early, or too quickly, the elderly person's physical and mental health is likely to suffer. People dealing with the elderly need to be particularly careful when assessing their needs and not put physical needs as a priority. There should, naturally, also be a spirit of self-advocacy where the elderly person is given as much responsibility as possible for their own well-being, depending on their mental and physical condition.

Safety in and around the home

Ageing brings about a gradual deterioration in the senses, and in balance, co-ordination and mobility which means that the elderly are more likely to suffer from accidents in the home. The following is a list of possible accidents that may occur:

- they are more likely to be injured or killed by falls in the home than any other age group
- forgetfulness can mean that the gas is left on, food is left to burn, cigarettes left alight, etc.
- loss of sensory perception may mean they cannot smell gas or smoke or see and hear potential hazards
- a reduction in balance and co-ordination means that, once they do start to fall, they are unable to save themselves
- brittle bones means that bones are more likely to break and take longer to heal

A great deal of home safety applies to all age groups. The following are some basic guidelines to home safety:

- everywhere should be well lit
- rugs should be non-slip and lie flat; floors should preferably have a fitted carpet so there are no edges to trip up on
- floors should not be polished
- flexes and wires should not trail on the floor
- electrical and gas appliances should be serviced and checked by approved tradesmen
- things should not be stored at height
- the bathroom should be adapted if necessary
- safe forms of heating should be used and free-standing paraffin stoves, calor gas heaters and so on should be avoided
- doors and windows should be secure and the front door should have a safety chain fixed on and, preferably, a spy hole so that the elderly person can see who is calling
- food hygiene is important as the elderly are less resistant to food poisoning bacteria; kitchens should be easy to clean and have a fridge and hygienic refuse disposal
- fire precautions need to be followed carefully, for example:
  (i)   all fires should be guarded

  (ii) the materials used in the furniture should be checked; they may be highly inflammable
  (iii) wiring should be checked every ten years
  (iv) sockets should not be overloaded
  (v)   cigarettes should not be smoked in bed
- in the garden the elderly should use garden tools with extended handles so they do not have to bend so far; this is a safer way to work

Health screening

Preventive medicine is a means of preventing illness before it it happens rather than treating the symptoms once they have appeared. Preventive medicine includes vaccination and inoculation, teeth and eye check-ups, X-rays, medical examinations and cervical smears. This service is provided by the NHS or private schemes to detect and prevent problems, but there is a great deal we can do for ourselves by living a healthy lifestyle. The following is a brief guide to the health checks available through the NHS or private schemes:

- chest X-rays should be taken every year to check the health of the lungs
- dental check-ups should be performed every six months to check the teeth and gums; dentures should be checked for comfort and fit every three years
- eye tests should be taken every year to check vision and to check that an eye disease such as glaucoma (see p. 16) is not developing
- a cervical smear should be taken every year as cervical cancer can develop rapidly; this provision does, however, vary from area to area
- a complete medical, checking blood pressure, heart rate, weight, brain and internal organs, is not usually available free of charge under the NHS, but can be paid for privately
- blood pressure should be checked every year

It is a fact that many people wait until they are showing the symptoms of a disease before they go to a doctor and this can sometimes be too late. Preventive health measures can do a great deal to give the elderly a healthier old age.

Sleep

Sleep is vital in order to allow the body to repair itself. The brain sends growth hormones into the bloodstream and these help the brain and body tissues to regenerate and repair themselves. Patterns of sleep vary throughout life and from person to person.

Babies and children need more sleep as their bodies are growing, whereas adults can exist on 6–8 hours sleep a night. The majority of research concludes that the elderly need less sleep, although there are some studies that do not agree with this view. However, although they may need less sleep, they also tend to worry about not sleeping properly and this anxiety can affect their sleep.

There are two types of sleep: first we fall into a deep sleep and about 1½–2 hours later we enter a lighter phase of sleep when we dream — this phase is called 'rapid eye movement' (REM) sleep (see Fig. 8.1). The elderly tend to have less deep sleep and, consequently, feel less refreshed the next day. The following are some of the factors that may affect the sleep patterns of the elderly:

- minor or major health disorders that prevent falling asleep, or staying asleep, e.g., anxiety and depression and stomach disorders
- needing to empty bladder in the night
- catnapping during the day
- lack of exercise
- drinking tea or coffee late at night (they are stimulants)
- eating less digestible foods late at night (these foods vary according to the individual)
- going to bed hungry
- an uncomfortable bed
- lack of ventilation
- drinking alcohol in the evening which makes the sleep that follows less refreshing

Insomnia, the inability to sleep, tends to increase with age, although it has been found that people often sleep for longer than they admit to. Everyone has a bad night's sleep sometimes, and it can be very frustrating. However, there are steps that can be taken to help ensure a reasonable night's sleep:

- as much exercise as possible should be taken during the day, depending on the person's state of health
- reading a good book or watching a relaxing television programme before going to bed
- a warm, milky drink rather than tea or coffee should be drunk as a nightcap
- the person should not be too hot or too cold
- the bed should be comfortable
- the bedroom should be kept well-ventilated

If the elderly person need less sleep, they need to have a positive attitude towards sleep. They are unlikely to be able to sleep the same hours they did when they were younger, so lying in bed, wide awake, in the early hours hoping to go to sleep is really a waste of time, and causes stress and anxiety. If the elderly person finds they are wide awake, feeling frustrated, then they should get up and, for example, make a drink and read until they feel relaxed and sleepy. The change of scene helps the tension to go and they are more likely to sleep when they get back to bed. Unfortunately, the greatest cause of insomnia is expecting not to sleep, and that attitude has to be changed by the person themselves. Once they realise that they can use the wakeful time positively, insomnia ceases to be such a threat. Sometimes the insomnia becomes so bad that sleeping pills are prescribed, although this should only be a last resort. The problems with sleeping pills are:

- they tend to last into the next day, and the person may find it difficult to concentrate

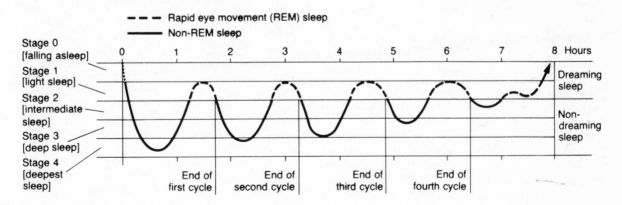

Fig. 8.1 The sleep cycle.

- sleep patterns are affected, and can take up to two months to return to normal after a course of sleeping pills; sleeping pills reduce the periods of rapid eye movement sleep and the intensity of dreams
- the quality of sleep is diminished and is not so refreshing
- there can be side-effects after using them for a week or two, e.g., indigestion, loss of appetite, rashes and, especially for the older elderly, confusion
- dependency may develop within a few weeks, and insomnia frequently gets worse when the course of sleeping pills stops

Personal needs

Everyone has personal needs and if these are satisfied self-confidence and self-esteem are improved. The elderly have the same personal needs as most people.

- *The need to feel wanted*   A feeling of being useless and good for nothing may occur in old age, especially at retirement. Confidence can be shattered by a feeling that friends, family and workmates no longer need you.
- *The need to feel attractive*   People who have taken care in their appearance throughout life will continue to do so into old age; this improves self-esteem.
- *The need to have control of our own lives*   Dependency puts the person who is being cared for at a disadvantage if they believe they are in an inferior position. One of the skills of a good carer is to be able to help the elderly person cope with their problems yet still encourage independence as far as possible in other areas of their life.
- *The need to have someone to care for and love*   Sometimes this is not possible, but even caring for a pet can be beneficial. When an animal or person relies on you, you feel needed and there is more of a purpose to life.

The carer should bear these needs in mind at all times. It is very easy when faced with caring for the elderly to cater only for their physical needs and forget their psychological needs. It is easy to understand why this happens because, generally, residential homes, day centres, hospital wards, etc., are understaffed and it takes the carers all their time to do the everyday tasks of toileting, washing, dressing, feeding and so on; there is little time left for talking at leisure. For the elderly living alone there is sometimes very little human contact, and there is the risk of isolation and loneliness. This problem is reduced for the elderly living as a couple, or for the elderly who live with their family, although in some cases many of their needs are ignored by others too busy to spend time with them.

Summary of keypoints

- The healthy eating guidelines of cutting down on salt, sugar and fats and increasing the intake of fibre applies to everyone, including the elderly. Unless the elderly person has a digestive problem, they can follow a normal diet.
- Exercise is beneficial to the elderly and improves the circulation, lung capacity, muscles, bones and joints. An exercise programme should not be started without consulting a doctor.
- Leisure activities are a good means of relaxation, but health, time availability and finances need to be taken into consideration.
- Sound financial advice and budgeting are important in old age because, statistically, the elderly are more likely to be on the poverty line. Poverty can affect the physical and mental health of a person.
- Retirement should be viewed in a positive rather than a negative light. Advanced planning for retirement can help the elderly person develop a positive attitude.
- Satisfying and fulfilling personal relationships are just as important for the elderly yet society, in general, seems to give this area little consideration.
- Care should be taken over the type and suitability of housing for the elderly. The elderly spend a higher proportion of their time at home and well-planned accommodation can help them to maintain their independence.
- Safety in the home is vital as many of the elderly have deteriorating senses and are therefore more likely to suffer from accidents in and around the home.
- Health screening tests are often able to detect a health problem before the symptoms are felt. Early treatment can, therefore, prevent a health problem from developing.
- The elderly have the same personal requirements as the rest of the population and they need to feel wanted, loved and attractive, as well as needing to feel they have control over their own lives. These needs should be uppermost in the minds of those dealing with and caring for the elderly.

Assignments

1. Ask a community dietician (contact the local hospital for details) to come and visit your group to talk about the dietary needs of the elderly. The following are some points you may like to cover:

- common misconceptions
- how the dietary needs of the elderly may differ from those of the rest of the population
- coping with special diets
- what local provision there is, e.g., help and advice, information sheets, home visits and so on
- facts about the local meals-on-wheels service; price, quality and who uses the service

2. Find out the type of exercise classes available for the elderly in your area; include who runs them, the cost and whether they are well-attended.

3. Invite a physiotherapist to talk to your group about the exercise needs of the elderly. The following are some points you may like to include:

- exercise for the average healthy older person
- the different needs of the age groups 60–70, 70–80, 80 +
- special exercise programmes for the elderly with health problems

4. The leisure interests of the elderly are not limited to the stereotypes of knitting and gardening. List some leisure interests that would be suitable for the following types of elderly people.

- A recently retired couple with adequate finances and good health looking for something different and exciting. Willing to commit evenings and weekends.
- A 75-year-old widow living in a ground floor flat. She has mild arthritis and a limited amount of money. Would like to meet other people, but not just other elderly widows. Has always been good with her hands.
- An elderly couple with a supportive family, yet living independently. They would like to do something that involves thought.
- A variety of pastimes to interest a group of elderly people attending a day centre once a week. The leisure interests need to be able to run on a low cost budget and should cater for those with a variety of abilities and health problems.

5. Check that you understand the meanings of these terms:

- Contributory Pension Scheme
- Non-contributory Pension Scheme
- Means Testing

Research briefly into the history of the financial welfare support of the elderly in Great Britain since the turn of the century. Include the following in your research:

- The poor-law and the workhouse
- Old Age Pensions Act, 1908
- Widows, Orphans and Old Age Contributory Pensions Act, 1925
- Poor-law Act, 1930
- Assistance Board; introduced in response to needs arising from the war years (1939–45)
- Beveridge Report, 1942
- Social Security Pensions Act, 1975

6. Find out about pre-retirement courses in your area. These may be run by:

- local Education Authority (community education section)
- county councils for their employees
- the forces (for their members who intend to retire early)
- industry and the private sector

Try and arrange to speak to one or more of the people concerned with organising and/or running these courses and ask what they believe are the key points to be conveyed about retirement.

7. Speak to elderly members of your family who have retired and ask them how they feel about retirement. You may wish to cover the following areas:

- their own attitudes towards retirement.
- how they feel society sees them, e.g., loss of status, etc.
- financial situation
- changes they would like to see introduced by the Government
- advice they would give people about to retire

8. Find out about the ways other societies and faiths regard both marriage and old age. For example, in India widows are not allowed to remarry, although widowers are. You may like to include:

- India; both Hindus and Moslems
- Islamic countries, e.g., Iran
- China
- The Mormons (based in Salt Lake City, USA)

9. As a group, comment on the following people's personal relationships:

STAFFS UNIVERSITY LIBRARY

- elderly couple in their 60s
- elderly couple in their 80s
- widower of 70
- widow of 70
- unmarried woman of 65
- unmarried man of 65

10.   Discuss the differing needs and priorities of relationships in these age groups:

- under 16
- 16–20
- 20–30
- 30–40
- 40–60
- 60 +

Remember not to use stereotypes.

11.   Much research has been carried out about sexuality in the older person and the results seem to suggest that society has many misconceptions about the sex lives of older people. Try and obtain copies of some of the following reports to find out the conclusions they reach:

- Kinsey (1948 and 1953)
- Masters and Johnson (1966)
- Shere Hite ('The Hite Report' published by Corgi)

12.   One of the major problems facing a relationship is when one of the partners retires. Contact your local Relate counsellor (previously the Marriage Guidance Council) and ask if she/he would talk to your group about the type of problems the over 60-year-old may have in a relationship.

13.   Certain health problems may mean that a couple have to adapt their sex life. Consider the way any of the following problems may affect a couple's sex life:

- heart disease
- bone diseases, e.g., arthritis
- high blood pressure
- a stroke
- diabetes

If you have difficulty finding information, perhaps a doctor or nurse dealing with the elderly may be able to help.

14.   Look at the changes in the family on page 55 and discuss how far you think they affect the way the elderly population is cared for. Do you feel elderly relatives are the responsibility of the family?

15.   Discuss the role of grandparents, and list the points you have made. Also consider any problems that might cause conflict such as over-interference, spoiling grandchildren, and so on.

16.   The Income Support system is very complex, and many elderly people may have situations which make the assessment of their benefits complicated. Obtain a copy of *A Guide to Income Support* (SB20) which briefly outlines the various benefits available, and indicates which leaflets to read for further information about each benefit.

17.   Isolation, desolation and loneliness are all likely to increase in old age. When dealing with the elderly, what factors do you think should be considered in order to encourage social contact? You may wish to include:

- the various different situations of the elderly
- their needs, e.g., what they want for themselves
- their wants, e.g., if they do not want to be sociable how far should we encourage them
- the type of provision that would be suitable for their needs

18.   As a group, discuss housing for the elderly.

- Should the elderly be encouraged as far as possible to stay in their own homes (by the help of grants, aids, adaptations, support agencies and domiciliary services) for as long as possible?
- Should warden-controlled, sheltered housing be more readily available? Should it be council or privately funded?
- Should there be a comprehensive housing scheme introduced to cater for all the needs of the elderly, i.e., as they become less independent should they move on to the next stage of housing?

19.   Design suitable and practical living accommodation for:

- an elderly and fairly immobile widow
- a widower, reasonably healthy, but needing company
- a residential home for the elderly

20.   Arrange a visit to the Disabled Living Foundation, 346 Kensington High St, London W14 8NS to look at the types of equipment and adaptations available for the elderly disabled for the home and garden.

21.   Write a set of home safety guidelines for the elderly under the following headings:

- fire
- prevention of falls

- electrical safety
- gas safety
- kitchen safety
- bathroom safety
- security

22.   Find out about the health check-ups available to the elderly in your area. Include the following tests:

- X-ray
- mammography
- rectal examination
- breast examination
- cervical smear
- complete medical check-up
- blood test
- blood pressure
- eye test
- dental check-up

Find out:

- how often the check-ups are carried out
- whether the person pays, i.e., private or NHS provision
- whether a recall system operates
- whether referral is from a doctor or by self

23.   Find out the average number of hours' sleep needed by:

- a newborn baby
- a toddler
- a 10-year-old
- a 16-year-old
- an adult
- an elderly person

24.   As a group, discuss what you think are the basic human psychological and emotional needs. Discuss how society can ensure that the elderly, whether living alone, as a couple, with their family, in sheltered accommodation or in a residential home, have these needs met.

9

CARE OF THE ELDERLY PATIENT

Caring for an elderly patient may be on a short- or long-term basis. Sometimes what is initially thought to be a short-term illness may develop into something more long-term because of unexpected complications. The patient's needs must, therefore, be constantly assessed and reassessed.

The elderly patient may be cared for in any one or more of the following situations:

- in their own home by their spouse, family and/or friends
- in their own home by the domiciliary services
- in the home of their family by their family
- in the home of their family who are also helped by the domiciliary services
- in a nursing home
- in hospital

In any nursing situation the patient's medical, emotional, physical and social needs should be the major concern of the carer, whether the carer is medically qualified, part of the family, or a friend. These needs change frequently, and the carer needs to be aware of this and be willing to reassess the situation and seek advice if necessary.

The nursing process

A fairly recent development in nursing care is the introduction of what is called the nursing process. This approach sees nursing as a complete whole, rather than a series of separate tasks, and this idea of a nursing continuum helps to make the patient the key figure in the assessment. The nursing process, although geared to qualified nurses, can help all people caring for elderly patients gain insight into good nursing techniques.

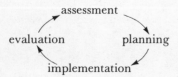

The idea behind this approach is to avoid the type of nursing based on treating the disease rather than the individual. Each individual patient has different needs, even if they are suffering from the same disease, and the nursing process acknowledges this fact.

The following is a brief explanation of the nursing process approach.

- *Assessment* usually takes place in the patient's home, unless they are an emergency admission to hospital. Assessment may be made by the community nurse, health visitor or GP, for example, and the patient's past history can be found out by asking the patient or, if this is not possible, the relatives.
- *Planning* is working out exactly what type of nursing care the patient needs. The decision is ideally made in consultation with the patient and his or her family.
- *Implementation* of these plans is more than just physical nursing care; it is also encouraging and motivating the patient to be as independent as possible.
- *Evaluation* needs to be an ongoing process to check that the care given is achieving the goals set and, if not, altering the planning.

This nursing process applies to the patient at home and in hospital.

Before going on to look at the nursing of elderly patients in the home and in hospital, it would be useful to be aware of some of the qualities of a good nurse/carer.

- Seeing the patient as an individual with a health problem rather than as a series of symptoms to be treated.
- An awareness of the patient's need for dignity and privacy at all times.
- Insight into the patient's emotionally vulnerable state. The patient will probably be more likely to become depressed, anxious and introspective because they are not well.

- The need to promote as much independence as possible, yet offer adequate support when required.
- The ability to give genuine loving care.
- Respect for the patient.

This list is by no means complete, but is a starting point to make the carer aware of exactly what is required of them.

Home nursing

Nursing the elderly patient at home has many advantages: the patient and carer will probably have had time to build up a relationship so, ideally, communication will be better; the carer will know the patient's background and personality and the patient will be more relaxed about communicating his/her needs. The majority of invalids prefer to be nursed in the familiar home environment, and the elderly are no exception.

Nursing the elderly at home is not easy, especially over a long period of time. Support from the professional health services is vital, offering either medical advice or help and support to the carer. Taking on too much does not help the patient or the carer as she/he is likely to become overstressed and less able to cope. The following are some simple guidelines for the carer.

- The carer should use the local GP and health visitor as they will be able to talk through problems, offer practical help with nursing care and home adaptations, etc., and will also arrange for additional domiciliary help if it is needed.
- The carer should not forget his/her own needs; a healthy diet, exercise and rest are vital.
- The carer should keep up their own social life as far as possible.
- The caring should be shared with the family, friends and professionals when possib'e.

The qualities of a good nurse discussed on page 64 can easily be translated into practical nursing approaches for the carer at home.

1. *The patient as an individual* A patient still has the same needs as a well person. They need to be included in the preparation of their nursing programme, and time should be spent talking and explaining things to them. They must not feel a victim of their ill-health.

2. *The need for dignity and privacy* All too frequently, ill-health leads to a loss of privacy and dignity. Although this is more likely to happen in hospital wards, the home nurse should be aware of the need to allow privacy, particularly when dressing, undressing and toileting is involved. The patient should be consulted as to what suits them best. In the acutely and terminally ill there will, however, be an inevitable reduction of privacy if the patient needs a catheter or bedpan, for example. Generally, privacy can be found by encouraging people to knock before entering the sick room.

3. *The patient's emotional state* Ill-health makes everyone feel vulnerable, and the elderly especially because they are less able to cope with stressful situations. If an elderly patient is bedridden, or confined to one room, there is very little to do. The elderly patient will, therefore, have plenty of time to think about his/her health which may cause stress and lead to a state of depression and anxiety which makes nursing very difficult. There is no set answer to this problem but, again, encouraging independence is vital as is talking through any problems the patient may have. Depression and anxiety are more likely if the patient loses touch with reality. Encouraging contact with the outside world via visitors, the television, newspapers and books can help, unless the patient is very ill.

4. *Independence* Unless told otherwise by a doctor, the elderly patient should be as active as possible. It may be quicker to do things for the patient, but it is far better to encourage them to do things for themselves. Problems do arise when some carers believe they are being helpful by doing everything for the patient, but to remove the patient's independence is to remove their self-respect and autonomy and may even delay recovery.

5. *Loving care* Not everyone is able to offer the type of care needed to nurse someone who is very ill. There may be a variety of reasons for this, but the situation needs to be assessed objectively to decide what is in the best interests of the patient and the carer. People with doubts about their ability to nurse an elderly patient should talk to a doctor and/or health visitor, and the elderly person's family before making any decisions. It is important to explain what is happening to the patient, as research has shown that the patient would rather cope with the fact that a carer feels unable to offer the type of nursing care demanded than feel rejected because no explanation has been offered.

6. *Respect for the patient* This section is linked to treating the patient as an individual. There are fewer problems in this area in home nursing as, hopefully,

respect will already exist in the relationship between the carer and the patient. Respect is shown in how a person is treated physically and mentally; it is considering their feelings and the carer imagining themselves in the position of the patient. Although this may not come naturally, it is worth making the effort for the patient's benefit. The carer who is aware of the patient's individual needs will be better equipped to deal with the day-to-day nursing care.

Everyday nursing care in the home

The medical needs of the patient will have been assessed by their GP and any medication and treatment will be explained to the carer. Obviously, there is a vast range of illnesses that may affect the elderly including:

- short or long-term infections
- short or long-term effects of falls or injuries
- convalescence after a stay in hospital because of illness, injury or operation
- long-term degenerative diseases
- cancer

All these illnesses demand a different approach to nursing care and these approaches should be explained to the carer by the doctor, health visitor and/or district nurse. There are, however, some basic principles of home nursing which are pretty general in their application.

The sick room

The position of the sick room depends on the type and length of the illness. Short-term patients usually use their own bedroom as they recover quite quickly, whereas patients with long-term or degenerative illnesses have different considerations. The long-term sick room will need:

- easy access to the bathroom so that the patient can visit for themselves, or for the carer to empty commodes or bedpans and for washing facilities
- the patient may prefer to be near the everyday life of the home and, therefore, not feel so isolated
- ease of access should be considered for the wheelchair-bound
- it should be a pleasant environment as the long-term patient may be there for months, or even years. There should be plants, pictures, ornaments, etc., to look at, and a television and radio within easy reach. Flowers and plants should be taken out of the room at night as they remove vital oxygen from the air

In general, the sick room (see Fig. 9.1) should be:

- well-ventilated, but not draughty, with an average temperature of 60°–65°F (15.5°–18.3°C)
- well-lit for reading and medical treatment
- quiet
- arranged so that the bed is easily reached from both sides and away from draughts
- provided with chair/s for the patient and/or visitors
- equipped with a bedside table with a reading light, water, tissues, etc.
- equipped with some means of communication such as a bell, buzzer or intercom
- kept free of drugs as there is the danger of the patient taking a deliberate or accidental overdose

For any reasonably long-term illness, there are certain pieces of equipment that will be needed regularly. The equipment varies depending on the illness, so the following checklist is therefore only a suggestion.

1. *Personal hygiene*
- *Washing equipment* This should never be shared and should be kept on a tray, for example, so it can be brought to the bedside. Washing equipment may include:
  (i)   a bowl
  (ii) mild soap
  (iii) a soft flannel
  (iv) a towel
  (v)   a toothbrush, toothpaste, toothmug and mouthwash
  (vi) toiletries such as talcum powder, deodorant, cream and moisturiser, make-up, shaving equipment, shampoo, hairbrush and comb, nail scissors, file and brush. A hairdrier should be kept close at hand

2. *For convenience*
- kitchen roll
- moistened disposable tissues
- cotton wool
- polythene bags for rubbish disposal
- tissues

3. *Bedding* This should be made of a material that is easily washed and dried and should include:

- at least two bottom sheets, preferably fitted for ease of bedmaking
- about four pillows to support the back when sitting up
- a duvet, or blankets if the patient prefers

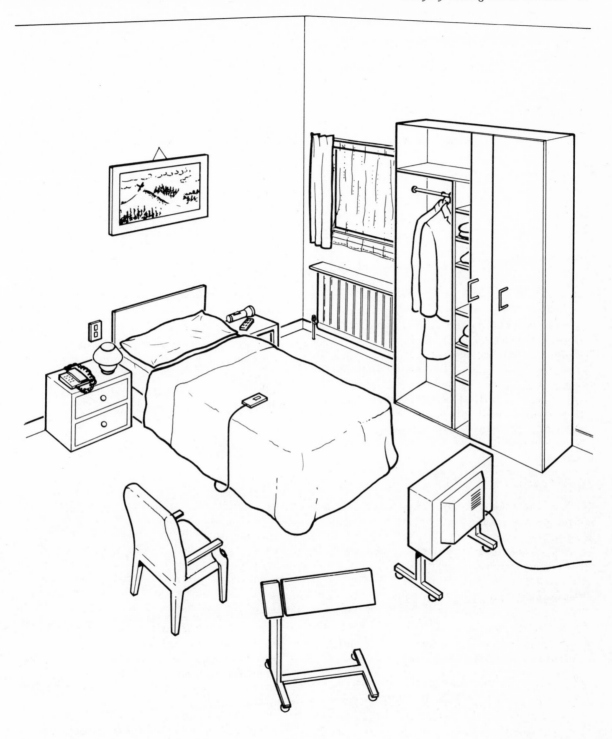

Fig. 9.1 The sick room.

- a plastic bedcover if there is a risk of incontinence

4. *Clothing*

- change of night clothes ⎫
- bedjacket or cardigan   ⎬ all easily washable
- dressing gown   ⎭
- slippers
- bedsocks

5. *Useful equipment*

- bedpan, urinal or commode
- a bedtable
- backrest
- continence aids
- thermometer

Care of the sick room

It is likely that the sick room will be occupied for most of the day by the patient so it may become stuffy and dusty from the bedding. It is far more pleasant for the patient to be in a clean and fresh-smelling room, and cleanliness helps to stop the spread of infection. Planning the cleaning depends on the carer and the patient. If the patient is mobile, they may leave the room to have a bath or sit in another room while the room is cleaned and the bed made. If they are very sick or terminally ill, the cleaning should be done as quietly as possible so that they are not disturbed.

A general routine for cleaning the sick room for a mobile patient would be:

- a general tidy up, i.e., throwing away old tissues, magazines, newspapers, etc., and emptying the bin
- replacing water and bringing a clean glass
- opening windows for ventilation
- vacuuming the carpet
- dusting surfaces, preferably using either a spray polish or damp cloth so that the dust does not rise
- wiping over washable surfaces with disinfectant

If the patient is bed bound, there are different considerations:

- because vacuum-cleaning may be noisy for the patient a carpet cleaner can be used instead
- there may be a commode to empty and clean

As the patient will spend a great deal of time in the sick room, minor considerations should be made as small details may easily niggle the patient. A draughty window, a crooked picture, books out of reach and so on become very irritating; so everything should be geared towards the comfort of the patient. The patient should be consulted about any changes as the carer should not be so busy tidying and cleaning that they forget to include the patient.

The sick bed

Because of the time spent in bed, the sick bed needs to be comfortable. The ideal sick bed should:

- be a single bed so there is easy access from both sides
- have a firm and level mattress. If the mattress is not firm, a board can be put underneath it. It is easier to give bedpans and wash the patient if the mattress is firm and it is more comfortable for sleeping on
- be higher than the average bed; preferably about 71–76 cms (2 feet 4 inches–2 feet 6 inches) high. If it is lower, bed making becomes difficult and the carer may damage their back. If it is higher, the patient will find it difficult to get out of bed

If the patient is incontinent, the mattress should have a waterproof sheet covered with a drawsheet. The sheets should be made of a polyester/cotton mixture for easy washing and drying. If the bed needs raising, it is possible to improvise by using wooden blocks, bricks or chairs.

Bed making

Bed making is a task that will need to be done more than once a day if the patient spends all day in bed. There is nothing worse than an uncomfortable bed with rumpled sheets and for the elderly immobile patient there is the added risk of bedsores developing. Bed making is obviously easier if the patient is not in the bed, but this is not always possible. There are two methods of bed making suggested and it is a good idea if the following guidelines are taken into consideration:

- the clean sheets and pillowcases should be collected together beforehand
- a binbag should be kept at hand in case the bed linen is heavily soiled
- work carefully so as little dust as possible is raised
- the mattress, cover, sheet, waterproof sheet, etc., should be free from wrinkles
- fitted bottom sheets are easier to use otherwise the edges of flat sheets have to be mitred to prevent them becoming loose
- the top sheet should be high enough to reach the shoulders

- explain what is being done to the patient
- the carer should look after their back by following the guidelines for bed making in Fig. 9.2.

Bed making when the patient is in bed is easier with two people, but this is not always possible. The following instructions have been written with one person in mind.

- Two chairs should be placed back-to-back at the end of the bed as these can be used to put the bedclothes on.
- All the bedclothes around the bed should be untucked.
- Each of the top covers should be removed one by one by folding them into thirds on the bed. The bottom of the cover should be moved two-thirds of the way up the bed and the top of the cover moved to meet the fold. The folded cover should be placed over the chairs.
- The patient should be left covered by the top sheet, and a blanket as well if they are cold.
- All the pillows except one should be taken away and the pillowcases taken off.

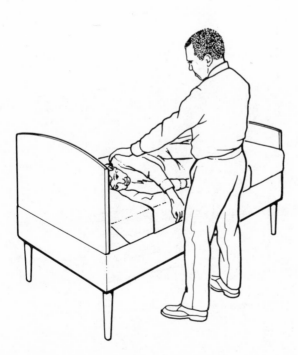

Fig. 9.2 Bed making. The back should be kept straight, knees bent, feet apart and comfortable non-slip shoes worn.

- The patient should be asked to roll on to their side on the other side of the bed from the carer. The carer should move the pillow for them or roll them over carefully if they are not able to roll over themselves.
- If there is a risk of the patient falling out of bed, a cotside should be used or chairs can be used to improvise with.
- Each piece of the bottom bed linen should be rolled up towards the patient's back (see Fig. 9.3).
- The mattress cover should be checked to see that it is straight.
- The half-rolled clean sheet should be placed beside the dirty rolled sheet and tucked in, mitring the edges if it is not a fitted sheet.
- A bottom sheet is mitred by:
  (i) tucking in the sheet at the foot of the bed
  (ii) lifting the side edge of the sheet about 45 cm (18 inches) from the bottom corner of the bed and tucking in the edge
  (iii) tucking the long edge of the sheet in
- If a plastic sheet is being used on top of the bottom sheet, it should be unrolled over the clean sheet.
- If a drawsheet is being used, it should be unrolled over the plastic sheet.
- The patient should be rolled towards the carer and over the rolls of bed linen. The pillows should be moved to make them comfortable, and the cotside too if it is being used.
- The carer should move to the other side of the bed.
- The remaining half of the dirty bed linen should be rolled up.
- The clean bottom sheet should be unrolled and tucked in and the edges mitred.
- The plastic sheet and drawsheet, if used, should be unrolled and tucked in (see Fig. 9.4).
- The patient should be moved on to their back and the pillows replaced. The pillowcase of the pillow that remained on the bed should be changed too.
- The topsheet should be replaced with a clean one if necessary, tucked in and the corners mitred. The sheet should have a tuck put in at the bottom to allow room for the patient to move their feet.
- When the patient is comfortable, and the dirty bed linen has been dealt with, the carer should wash their hands.

When two people are making a bed, one can hold the patient safely on his/her side while the other person deals with the bed making. Sometimes the patient may have a condition that makes it impossible for them to be left lying flat while the bed

STAFFS UNIVERSITY LIBRARY

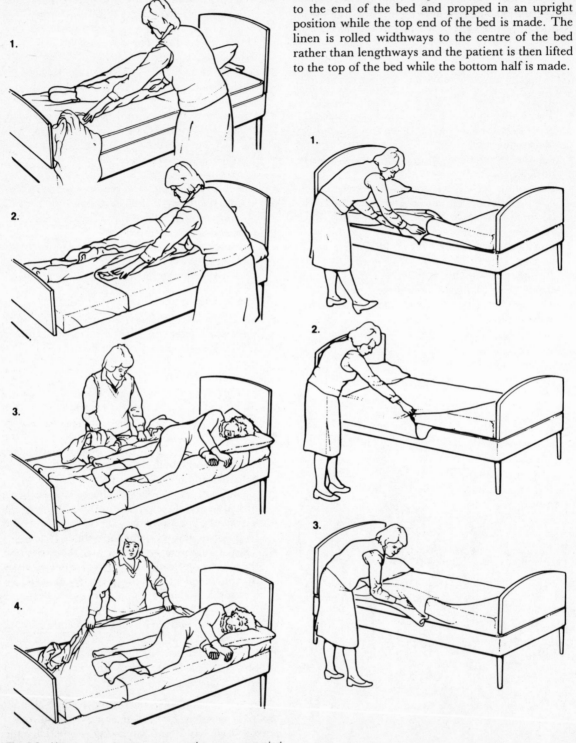

is made. In this case, the patient will need to be lifted to the end of the bed and propped in an upright position while the top end of the bed is made. The linen is rolled widthways to the centre of the bed rather than lengthways and the patient is then lifted to the top of the bed while the bottom half is made.

Fig. 9.3 How one person can make an occupied bed. **1.** The bed linen is rolled up. **2.** The clean linen is laid on one half of the mattress. **3.** The dirty linen is pulled through. **4.** The clean linen is unrolled.

Fig. 9.4 Positioning a plastic sheet and draw sheet.

Lifting and moving an immobile patient

In any long-term home nursing of a patient who is immobile or who finds it difficult moving around unsupported, there will be a certain amount of lifting involved. Books are not the ideal way of finding out how to lift; practical demonstrations by a local hospital physiotherapist or district nurse to help prevent the risk of back injury to the lifter are more informative. There is also equipment and adaptations available to borrow, hire or buy to help lift and move patients (see p. 45–7).

Before a patient is lifted, the following guidelines should be noted:

- work in pairs as this is easier and safer
- before a patient is lifted, find out exactly what should be done and, if necessary, an able-bodied person should be practised on
- what the carer should and should not do should be checked with the patient's medical staff
- what is being done should be explained to the patient and they can be told what they can do to help

Various lifting methods have been devised using either one or two lifters. The following are some examples of these lifts.

1. Lifting a patient up the bed from a flat position in pairs.
2. Lifting a patient up the bed from a flat position singlehanded.
3. Turning a helpless patient in bed in pairs.
4. Turning a helpless patient in bed singlehanded.
5. Moving a patient from the bed to a chair in pairs.
6. Moving a patient from the bed to a chair singlehanded.
7. Moving a patient from a sitting position to a standing position in pairs.
8. Moving a patient from a sitting position to a standing position singlehanded.

1. *Lifting a patient up the bed from a flat position in pairs* This lift should, ideally, be done in pairs unless the patient is light or is able to help. There are three ways to complete the lift: using a handgrip, using a drawsheet if there is one, or by using a shoulder lift.

Using a handgrip
  i The lifters face one another on opposite sides of the bed.
  ii The patient crosses his/her arms across his/her chest.
  iii The lifters grasp hands beneath the patient's

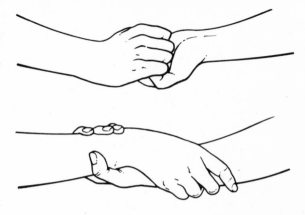

Fig. 9.5 Two methods of making a handgrip to move a patient up the bed.

thighs and behind the patient's back using one of the following handgrips; holding fingers or holding wrists (see Fig. 9.5 and Fig. 9.6).
  iv The lifters must keep their backs straight and knees bent with feet placed about 30 cm (12 inches) apart.
  v The lifters lift together moving the patient up the bed by transferring their weight on to the foot nearest the top of the bed.

Using a drawsheet
  i The lifters face one another on opposite sides of the bed.
  ii The patient crosses his/her arms across his/her chest.
  iii The drawsheet is untucked.
  iv The lifters grip the drawsheet near the patient's thighs and behind the buttocks, as close to the patient as possible.
  v The lifters lift together, supporting the patient's back with the forearm closest to the top of the bed, moving the patient up the bed by transferring their weight on to the foot nearest the top of the bed.

The shoulder lift
  i The lifters put a shoulder under the patient's armpits.
  ii The lifters grasp hands under the patient's thighs using the finger or wrist grip (see Fig. 9.7).
  iii The lifter's other hand is put flat on the bed.
  iv The lifters lift together moving the patient up the bed by transferring their weight on to the foot nearest the top of the bed.

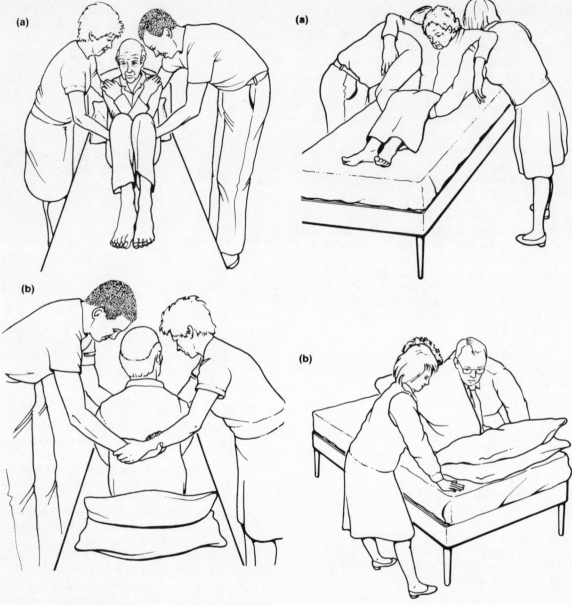

Fig. 9.6 Position of lifters using a handgrip (**a**) From the front. (**b**) From the back.

Fig. 9.7 Shoulder lift (**a**) From the front. (**b**) From the back.

2. *Lifting a patient up the bed from a flat position singlehanded* It is possible to use the shoulder or underarm lift if the patient is able to help.

Shoulder lift The lifter puts his/her shoulder under the patient's arm and holds the patient's thigh. As the lifter lifts, the patient pushes on the bed with their free arm and leg (see Fig. 9.8).

Underarm lift The patient links arms with the lifter, holding on to their shoulder while the lifter holds the patient's shoulder. The patient bends their knees and pushes on the bed with their feet and their free hand as the lifter lifts (see Fig. 9.9).

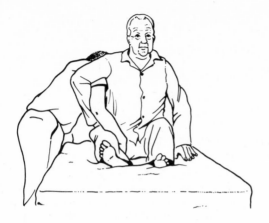

Fig. 9.8 Shoulder lift single-handed.

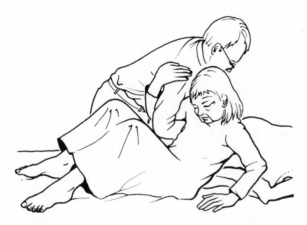

Fig. 9.9 Underarm lift single-handed.

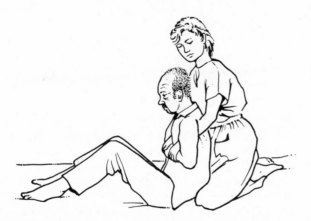

Fig. 9.10 Moving a helpless patient single-handed.

If the patient is not able to help, the singlehanded lifter needs to work from on the bed. The pillows need to be moved away and the lifter kneels on the bed behind the patient. The lifter puts his/her arms under the patient's armpits and holds their forearms. As the patient is lifted he/she pushes on the bed with their feet if possible (see Fig. 9.10).

3. *Turning a helpless patient in bed in pairs* This is the best way of moving a helpless patient as two people can make the lift more smoothly. A helpless patient will need to be turned every two hours to prevent bedsores and will also have to be moved when the bed is being made.

i   The lifters face each other at opposite sides of the bed.
ii The bedclothes are pulled back and all but one of the pillows taken away.
iii The pillows are moved to one side of the bed.
iv The patient's right arm is put across his/her chest with the right arm down by their side and the right leg across the left (see Fig. 9.11, 1.).
v   The lifter on the left-hand side of the bed pulls the patient on to his/her side by holding the shoulder with one hand and the buttocks with the other (see Fig. 9.11, 2.).
vi The lifter on the right-hand side helps by pushing the patient over gently.
vii The patient needs to be moved to the middle of the bed so they do not fall out. This is done by the lifters holding hands under the patient's buttocks and thighs and lifting.

If the patient needs support, a pillow can be put behind their back. To turn them again, the same instructions can be used reading left for right and vice versa (see Fig. 9.11, 3.).

4. *Turning a helpless patient in bed singlehanded*

i   The lifter stands by the bed.
ii The bedclothes are pulled back and all but one of the pillows taken away.
iii The pillows are moved to one side of the bed.
iv The patient's right arm is put across his/her chest with the right arm down by their side and the right leg across the left.
v   The lifter pulls the patient towards him/her by putting one hand on the patient's shoulder and the other hand on their buttocks. The pillows can be used for support, if necessary, and to prevent the patient rolling out of bed while they are being centred.

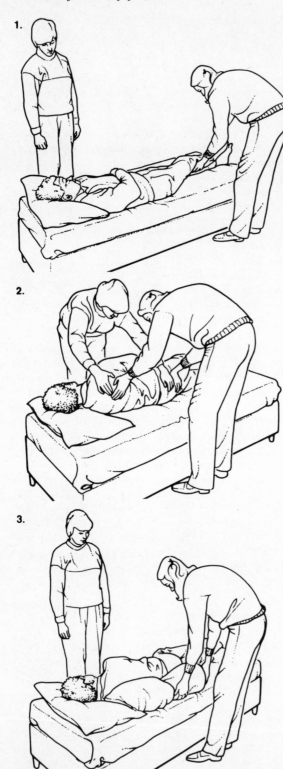

1.

2.

3.

Fig. 9.11   Turning a helpless patient in bed in pairs.

5.   *Moving a patient from the bed to a chair in pairs*
Someone who is bedridden, but not seriously ill, should be encouraged to spend some time sitting in a chair. Apart from the fact that it is a change of scene, it also helps reduce the likelihood of developing certain health disorders associated with lack of movement, e.g., pressure sores, deep vein thrombosis and muscle wastage. Before making the move, the following should be done:

- the chair should be put at right angles near the bed, preferably against the wall so it does not slide
- the patient should have non-slip footwear on
- the floor should be checked to make sure that there is nothing for the lifter or patient to slip on

Moving a patient from the bed to a chair in pairs if the patient is unable to stand unaided
   i   Both lifters stand on the same side of the bed as the chair.
   ii   The patient is helped to the edge of the bed.
   iii   Steps i–ii of the shoulder lift should be followed (see p. 71).
   iv   The patient is lifted evenly by the lifters straightening their knees.
   v   The patient is carried to the chair and lowered into it by the lifters bending their knees and holding on to the chair with their free hand.

Moving a patient back to bed from a chair
   i   The lifters help the patient towards the edge of the chair by bending their knees and holding hands under the patient's thighs.
   ii   The lifters put their shoulders under the patient's armpits and lift by straightening their knees, taking care to keep their back straight.

Moving a patient back to bed from a chair in pairs if the patient can stand
   i   The lifters face each other on the same side of the bed as the chair.
   ii   The patient moves to the edge of the bed and, if necessary, wedges his/her feet against the outside feet of the lifters to prevent slipping.
   iii   The lifters support the patient by his/her armpits and hands as he/she stands up.

6.   *Moving a patient from the bed to a chair singlehanded*

If the patient is unable to stand unaided   Because this lift is done by gently swinging the patient from the bed to the chair, the chair should have no arms. The chair should be facing the bed and close enough for the patient to swing round on to it.

   i   The lifter helps the patient to the side of the bed, making sure that the patient is wearing non-slip footwear.

ii The lifter wedges the patient's feet and knees against theirs and put the patient's shoulder nearest the top of the bed against their side.

iii The lifter holds the patient's elbow.

iv The lifter lifts the patient by shifting their weight on to their back leg.

v The lifter swings the patient round to the chair by shifting their weight to their other leg.

If the patient is able to stand The chair should be at right angles to the bed for this move.

i The patient is helped to the edge of the bed and their feet are placed on the floor.

ii The patient puts his/her hands on the lifter's shoulders and puts their head over the lifter's shoulder.

iii The lifter puts his/her arms under the patient's, supporting the upper back with the palms of their hands.

iv The lifter stands with knees bent and back straight with one foot inside the patient's feet.

v The lifter pushes up with their arms and shifts their weight on to their back leg.

vi The lifter shuffles sideways until the patient's legs are by the chair.

vii To sit the patient down, the lifter puts one leg in between the patient's legs, bends their knees, shifts their weight to their front leg, and gradually lowers the patient into the chair.

To get the patient back to bed, the moves are carried out in reverse order.

7. *Moving a patient from a sitting to a standing position in pairs* This move needs to be carried out when the immobile patient starts to walk again. The patient must be wearing non-slip footwear.

i The lifters stand close to the patient, one each side of the chair.

ii The patient can wedge his/her feet against the lifters' feet for stability.

iii The lifters put one arm under the patient's arm and the other on the chair, taking care that the chair does not tip over.

iv The lifters lift together, pulling the patient into an upright position by shifting their weight on to their back foot.

v The lifters use the arm that was holding the chair to support the patient's elbow.

8. *Moving a patient from a sitting to a standing position singlehanded*

i The lifter puts one leg in between the feet of the patient, and the other leg behind them.

ii The lifter holds each of the patient's elbows, getting the patient to hold the lifter's forearms.

iii The patient leans forward and the lifter pushes the patient's elbows up as the patient straightens their legs (see Fig. 9.12).

Moving a patient needs to be done in a sympathetic and caring way. The patient will probably be very aware of their loss of independence and mobility, and may feel guilty at the effort it takes to move them.

In most cases the patient will recover their mobility, so helping them in and out of bed and to a change of scene is a positive way of encouraging them to become mobile. For the elderly patient who is unlikely to recover their mobility, regular moving and lifting helps make them comfortable.

For the long-term disabled patient it is worthwhile finding out about the equipment and adaptations available. An outline of the type of equipment available to help the disabled maintain as much independence as possible in their everyday lives is found in Chapter 7.

Everyday care of the elderly patient

The standard of everyday care of the elderly patient can affect the rate of recovery. The patient may only need a little help or they may be dependent on the carer for almost all their personal needs. Either way, the standard of care needs to be high, with the patient's physical and mental comfort a priority. Some of the tasks the carer needs to do can be very embarrassing for the patient and they may feel a loss of dignity if they need to be given bedpans and washed by someone else. Sympathy and understanding on the part of the carer can help the patient feel more relaxed and the patient should never be left without means of communication for any length of time in case they need to summon help in an emergency.

Personal hygiene

Many patients are able to get to the bathroom with perhaps only the minimum amount of help. The less able will need to have their washing equipment (see p. 66) brought to the bedside and the very ill will need to be washed by a carer or nurse.

A patient should be washed twice a day unless told otherwise by a doctor. Washing has two benefits: firstly it makes the patient feel brighter and better and, secondly, any stale sweat and other waste products will be removed. Patients who use a bedpan

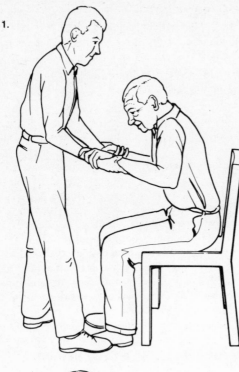

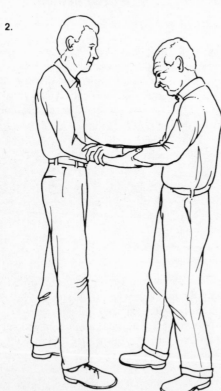

Fig. 9.12 Moving a patient from sitting to standing using the elbow grip.

or a commode should be able to wash their hands after use.

1.   *The patient who can wash themselves*   The patient may either strip wash, bath or shower, depending on their preference. If they bath or shower, a non-slip rubber mat is a useful safety measure to prevent slipping. Before the patient washes the following should be done:

- the bathroom should be warm enough
- the bath water should be the correct temperature (112°–120°F or 44°–49°C) or, if the patient is using the shower, it should be set in advance
- if necessary, the elderly patient should be helped to undress
- if they are able to bath alone, the door should stay unlocked
- if the elderly patient prefers, a plank can be put across the bath for them to sit on, or a chair can be put under the shower
- the bath, shower or sink should always be cleaned after use

Sometimes the elderly person may be embarrassed about being washed by someone else. Talking to them can help to ease any embarrassment.

2.   *The patient who can wash themselves in bed*

i   The washing equipment listed on page 66 should be brought to the bed and put on the bedside table.

ii   The bedclothes should be pulled back, but the patient left with a sheet to cover him/herself.

iii   If necessary, the patient should be helped to undress.

iv   A bowl should be ½ – ¾ filled with warm water.

The patient should be encouraged to wash alone, but they may need help to wash their back and buttocks.

3.   *The patient needing a bed bath*   As with all nursing processes, the equipment should be collected together beforehand. This includes:

- a bowl of warm water
- two flannels; one for the face and one for the body
- two small towels; one for the face and one for the body
- a large bath towel to put under the patient
- soap
- manicure equipment; nail scissors and nailbrush
- hairbrush and comb
- moisturising cream and make-up, etc., if required
- talcum powder

- hair washing equipment, if required
- teeth or denture cleaning equipment
- disposable wet wipes

Sometimes it is sensible to change the bed after a bed bath, therefore, all the bedmaking equipment should be collected together beforehand. The patient will also need clean nightclothes.

The routine will vary as the patient will not need to be manicured and hair washed everyday, but the following is the general pattern of bed bathing.

i If possible, the patient is put in an upright position on the bath towel. They should be covered with a sheet, with the rest of bedclothes pulled back, and undressed carefully.

ii The face, ears and neck should be washed with the face flannel. The patient should be asked to find out whether they usually use soap on their face.

iii The flannel should be rinsed in the bowl and used to rinse off the soap from the face, ears and neck.

iv The patient should be dried gently with the small towel.

v The patient's hands and arms should be washed, rinsed and dried, starting with the hands and working up to the armpits. If necessary, the fingernails should be cleaned.

vi The chest, abdomen and sides of the body should be washed.

vii The legs should be washed, rinsed and dried, separately, keeping the one that is not being washed covered up.

viii If talcum powder is used on the body, only a little should be used.

ix The patient is turned, using the technique shown on page 76, and their back washed, rinsed and dried.

x The genital region should be washed although many patients will do this for themselves. A separate flannel or, preferably, the disposable wet wipes should be used. Women are washed from front to back and with men it is important that the area beneath the foreskin is washed.

xi The buttocks and anal region should be washed using disposable wet wipes for washing the anus. Many patients prefer to wash the anal region for themselves.

4. *Care of the hands and feet* The fingernails should be cleaned and cut when necessary and toenails should be cut straight across to prevent problems such as ingrowing toenails developing. If there are

any problems or if cutting the nails is difficult, the advice of a chiropodist should be sought.

5. *Shaving* If a male patient is too unwell to shave themselves, the carer will need to do it everyday. An electric razor is easier, but this may not be an option if there is no socket nearby.

6. *Care of the hair* An invalid's hair soon gets out of condition so for the morale of the patient hair should be kept clean and brushed.

As with washing and bathing, the more able-bodied patient will be able to get to the bathroom to have his/her hair washed, and the sicker patient will need to have a hair wash in bed. For washing hair in bed, the following equipment should be collected together beforehand:

- a small, low stool or box
- a bowl of warm water
- a jug of warm water for rinsing but preferably two or three jugs to save going back to the bathroom
- shampoo and conditioner if necessary
- two plastic sheets
- two towels
- a brush and comb
- a hairdrier

Once the equipment has been collected together, the patient is prepared by wrapping one of the towels around their shoulders and laying them down across a pillow covered in a plastic sheet so that their head is over the edge of the bed. The other plastic sheet should be on the floor.

i The hair should be wetted carefully.

ii The hair should be shampooed and rinsed thoroughly.

iii If necessary, the jugs should be refilled to make sure that the hair is properly rinsed.

iv The hair should be dried with the other towel to remove excess water.

v The hairdrier is used to completely dry the hair.

vi When the hair has been washed and combed it should be arranged in the patient's usual style.

7. *Care of the mouth and teeth* If the patient has his/her own teeth they should be cleaned at least twice a day. The more able patient can clean their own teeth in the bathroom, but it is possible to clean teeth in bed. Equipment needed for this is:

- a toothbrush
- toothpaste
- a glass of water

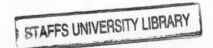
STAFFS UNIVERSITY LIBRARY

- a spitting bowl
- a tissue or towel to wipe the mouth

If possible, denture wearers should wear their false teeth otherwise their gums may shrink, they may find eating difficult and they may not appear at their best. If the patient can get to the bathroom, they should be able to clean their own dentures, otherwise the following equipment will need to be brought to the bed:

- a toothbrush
- denture cleaner
- a glass of water
- a spitting bowl
- a tissue or towel to wipe the mouth

Some illnesses affect the mouth making it dry, sore and crusted and possibly infected and the patient may have bad smelling breath. An unhealthy mouth is not only uncomfortable, it also affects the patient's ability to eat. The patient can, however, take preventive measures to help keep the mouth healthy which include:

- eating foods high in vitamins and other vital nutrients (see p. 49)
- drinking plenty of fluids
- regularly cleaning teeth or dentures

If the mouth does become unhealthy, the inside of the patient's mouth and the tongue can be cleaned by using a cotton bud dipped in either a sodium bicarbonate or a glycerin-thymol solution. After cleaning, the patient can rinse their mouth with an antiseptic mouthwash.

8.   *Care of the eyes*   The eyes should be cleansed carefully to remove any deposits that have built up in the corners. Cotton wool dipped in boiled, warm water can be used. The eyes should be wiped from the inside of the eye outwards, and the cotton wool discarded after each wipe.

9.   *Care of the nose*   Noses should be kept clean by blowing, and should not be poked around. A nose that is blown frequently may get sore, so vaseline can be used.

Elimination

The bed bound patient is usually very embarrassed and upset at having to use a bedpan or commode to pass urine and faeces. It needs a great deal of sympathy and understanding on the part of the carer to deal with the situation tactfully. A patient in bed is more likely to suffer from constipation either because of their diet, their illness, or because they are reluctant to use the bedpan or commode. Problems like this can be discussed with a district nurse or doctor.

The equipment

1.   *The male urinal*   This has a cap to put over the top to avoid spillage. The bed bound male patient should be sitting up when he is given the urinal. When he has finished, the urinal should be taken away, covered by kitchen roll or something similar, ready to be emptied. The patient's hands should be washed.

2.   *The female urinal*   This is easier to use than a bedpan and is smaller and lighter.

3.   *The bedpan*   Bedpans may be made of metal or plastic and are designed for men and women to defaecate in to. They can also be used for women to urinate into if they have no urinal (see Fig. 9.13).

4.   *The commode*   This is a chair with a bedpan fitted to the seat (see Fig. 9.14). Patients who can be moved prefer the commode to using bedpans and urinals.

5.   *The sanichair*   This is a wheelchair with a hole cut in the seat so the patient can be wheeled to the toilet and the chair positioned over the toilet seat. This gives additional independence.

The bedpan, urinal or commode should be cleaned and disinfected after use. It should then be rinsed and dried ready for reuse.

Some patients will have to be fitted with a catheter (a catheter is a thin, flexible tube inserted into the bladder to collect the urine). The tube is held in place by a small inflated balloon and the urine is collected

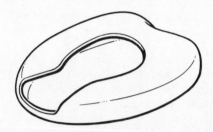

Fig. 9.13   The bedpan.

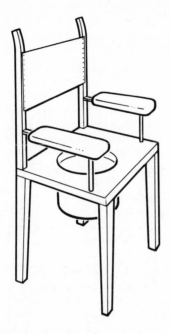

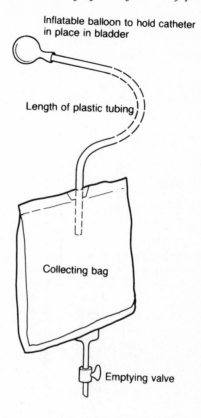

Inflatable balloon to hold catheter in place in bladder

Length of plastic tubing

Collecting bag

Emptying valve

Fig. 9.15 The urinary catheter.

Fig. 9.14 The commode has detachable armrests for ease of access.

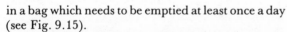

in a bag which needs to be emptied at least once a day (see Fig. 9.15).

Most carers will not be required to deal with catheters but, if they are, the process of emptying the catheter and dealing with the patient will be explained in detail by a nurse.

Patient comfort

Patient comfort is a vital element in recovery. This chapter has looked at the day-to-day aspects of patient care and the other factors affecting the patient will now be considered.

1. *Pressure sores* Any patient staying in bed and who is fairly immobile may develop pressure sores within a few days. Pressure sores are painful areas where the skin has broken and weeps fluid. Certain areas of the body are more prone to develop pressure sores than others (see Fig. 9.16). If left untreated, the sore develops into an ulcer and may become infected or gangrenous. The causes of pressure sores are:

- pressure and friction on the parts of the body where the bones are near the surface, e.g., buttocks, lower spine, elbows, knees, heels, ankles, shoulders, upper spine and hips; the sores are usually caused where these parts of the body touch the mattress
- chafing in places where the skin surfaces touch, e.g., the ankles, upper thighs, etc.
- scratching or rubbing in certain areas that may cause irritation

The problem will be exacerbated by the following factors:

- sweating
- bad circulation because of the illness or lack of movement
- incontinence
- skin in poor condition because of the illness or inadequate nutrition
- dirty and rumpled bedding

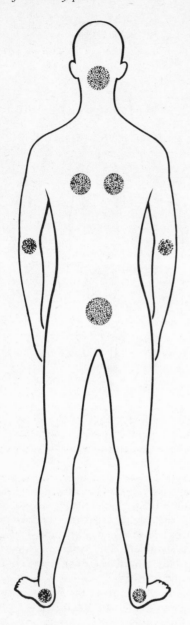

Fig. 9.16 Areas most likely to develop pressure sores.

- the bed should be made at regular intervals by smoothing the bedding and keeping it free from crumbs
- the patient should be kept clean
- the parts of the body most at risk from pressure sores need to be massaged to encourage circulation
- the patient should be on a well-balanced diet and given plenty of fluids to drink
- frequent use of the toilet, bedpan or commode should be encouraged. If the patient is incontinent any continence aids should be changed regularly
- an eye should be kept open for any signs that may suggest a pressure sore is developing
- sheepskins may be bought for the patient to sit or lie on
- bedclothes should be kept light
- a bedcradle can be used to keep the pressure of the bedclothes off the patient's body

2. *Exercise* The bedridden patient needs to do some form of exercise, however small, to help prevent joint stiffness, muscle wastage and deep vein thrombosis caused by poor blood circulation. Some simple exercises include circling the feet clockwise and anticlockwise, knee bends, lifting the legs, circling the hands and wrists and so on. More detailed exercises should be recommended by a district nurse or physiotherapist, depending on the patient's illness or disability.

3. *Rest and sleep* Rest and sleep are vital to us all as they give the body tissues an opportunity to repair and replenish themselves. The elderly invalid needs rest and sleep to recuperate but, ironically, it is usually more difficult to sleep during an illness. The carer can help to reduce the likelihood of insomnia by devising a simple and comforting bedtime routine based on the patient's own needs and wishes. For example, the patient who has always read a book before sleeping may want to continue to do so whilst others may prefer to watch television or do a crossword although, normally, a great deal depends on the extent of their illness. In general, a good bedtime routine will incorporate:

- helping the patient to use the toilet, bedpan or commode and washing their hands afterwards
- cleaning teeth or dentures
- pain relief if necessary. Pain may be caused by pressure sores, cold, joint aches, an uncomfortable bed, cramp and so on. Pain due to the illness will already be catered for in the patient's treat-

It is possible to prevent pressure sores developing if the following precautions are taken:

- the patient should change position at least every two hours; if the patient cannot do this unaided, the instructions on page 73 should be followed

ment but the home carer may need to alleviate some of the short-term types of pain mentioned above

- making the bed comfortable by, for example, straightening the sheets, raising or lowering pillows, etc.
- making sure the room is well-ventilated but not draughty
- checking that the patient has light, water, tissues, etc., and a means of communication nearby

Occasionally the elderly patient will develop insomnia (an inability to sleep). If the suggestions above do not work and the patient and the carer's health is being affected, a doctor may prescribe a course of sedatives (sleep-inducing drugs) on a short-term basis. There are, however, disadvantages in taking sedatives:

- the sleep induced by sedatives is different from normal sleep (see p. 59). The drugs work by slowing down the central nervous system so the sleep tends to be deeper and longer than usual and still affects the patient for some hours after they have woken up
- the drugs may lead to dependency because without them it may take some weeks to return to normal sleep patterns and there may even be withdrawal symptoms such as nightmares
- the sedatives do not deal with the underlying cause of insomnia

4. *Loss of appetite* Loss of appetite is very common during an illness. It may be temporary if the patient is going to recover, or it may be permanent if the patient is likely to die. The appetite usually diminishes with age, so any illness is likely to cause a loss of appetite. There are various factors to take into consideration when planning meals to stimulate the appetite. Perhaps one of the most important points is to not force the patient to eat the food either by too much persuasion, or by becoming upset if the food is left untouched. They cannot help their loss of appetite, and patience and good humour from the carer is helpful as it will not put pressure on the patient to eat.

Although much of this is common sense, the following are some guidelines for feeding the patient who has lost his/her appetite:

- the patient's food likes and dislikes should be found out; these may change on a day-to-day basis as ill health can make foods that the patient usually enjoys quite unappealing
- only small portions should be prepared as an

average-sized helping can be quite off-putting to an invalid

- the diet should be well-balanced with enough fibre to prevent constipation
- greasy, highly spiced or indigestible foods should be avoided
- food should be presented in an attractive way
- the patient should not be pressurised to eat, and they should be left to take their time
- the patient may like company when they eat, perhaps other members of the family may eat with them, or they may like to eat while watching the television
- any dietary instructions given by a doctor, dietician or nurse should be incorporated

Some patients may not be able to feed themselves in which case the carer will need to feed them. Being fed by someone can be a very humiliating experience for the patient: it is an acknowledgement that they are dependent on someone else and there is also the idea that babies are fed too, so they may feel as if they are in some sort of second childhood. The carer can help to minimize these feelings and, hopefully, the patient will recover sufficiently to feed themselves. The following are some guidelines for feeding patients:

- the patient should be comfortable, preferably propped upright so they can see the food. However, some may need to lie down on their side
- a bib should never be used; this is the ultimate insult and more likely to make them feel like helpless babies, a tea towel or napkin can be put around their shoulders
- the person feeding the patient needs to be comfortable
- the patient should be asked how they would like to eat. We all tackle a meal differently; some save the best to last, others eat the vegetables first and some may like it all mixed together. The patient should be offered the choice as this gives them some control over the meal
- the patient should be asked to find out whether they would like sips of drinks during the meal or afterwards, etc.
- the forkfuls of food should be timed; too fast and the patient may choke; too slow and they become bored
- the patient should be encouraged to feed themselves as soon as possible

There are special eating aids and adaptations available for the person who has difficulty using normal cutlery (see p. 46). It may be advisable to use these if it means the patient can feed themselves sooner.

5. *Observing the patient*　The carer has many roles. The way in which the home carer caters for the patient's physical, mental and emotional needs has been looked at, but she/he must also be aware of any changes in the patient's condition. The patient may not be aware of any changes him/herself so the carer needs to be vigilant. The simple ways of noting any changes in the patient's condition are by taking and keeping a record of temperature, pulse and respiratory rate.

- *Taking a temperature*　Usually, a patient's temperature is taken in the mouth unless the elderly patient is unconscious or confused. The thermometer records the temperature in degrees centigrade, but older thermometers may be in Fahrenheit. The thermometer should be stored in a jar of antiseptic solution if it is used regularly. The following are some guidelines to be aware of when using a thermometer.

  i The mercury should be shaken down to the bulb of the thermometer.

  ii The thermometer should be placed under the patient's tongue.

  iii It should be left in place for two minutes.

  iv It is then taken out the mouth, the bulb is wiped and a reading taken.

  v The result is recorded.

  vi The mercury should then be shaken back down into the bulb of the thermometer. .

  If the patient is unconscious or confused, their temperature has to be taken in the rectum. The rectal thermometer is different from the normal clinical thermometer and has a less pronounced bulb. It should be shaken as before and greased before it is inserted into the rectum. It should be held in place for two minutes, wiped clean, and a reading taken. The temperature reading is higher than that taken by mouth, and is usually 37°C (98.5°F). The normal temperature reading under the tongue is 36.9°C (98.4°F) although it should be stressed that temperature should not be relied upon as a measure of the degree of illness: the patient may be quite ill, but with no change in temperature.

- *Taking the pulse*　The pulse should be checked for rate, strength and rhythm. Rate is the number of times the heart beats per minute; strength is the power of the beat, whether strong, normal or weak; and rhythm is the regularity of the beat. The pulse is taken on the patient's wrist using the fingertips and not the thumb as the thumb has its own pulse which may be confusing. A watch with a second hand should be used for checking the pulse rate. An adult's pulse rate is between 60–80 beats a minute.

- *Checking the respiratory rate*　Inhaling, when the air is taken in and the chest cavity inflates, and exhaling, when the air is expelled and the chest cavity deflates, is one respiration. The average rate of respiration is 16–18 times a minute, but the patient may subconsciously alter this if he/she realises that respiration is being checked. It is best checked when the patient is either asleep or unaware of the fact that it is being taken.

General observation is the best way of telling whether the patient's condition has improved or deteriorated. A good carer will be aware of changes because of the relationship she/he has built up with the patient.

6. *Communication*　Communication is vital in all walks of life. It is a two-way process: we communicate our needs and wishes to the world around us, and perceive the needs and wishes of the people around us. The patient may find that communication becomes difficult during an illness for physical reasons, such as serious illness, stroke, etc., or because of their mental condition. The carer should be aware of these problems and give the patient the opportunity to express themselves, maybe using different means such as asking the patient a series of yes/no questions, or maybe using sign language or writing. The usual means of communication are:

- verbal and non-verbal (expression, position, etc., often called body language)
- written
- touch
- visual

All these means of communication can be used by the carer caring for the elderly patient. An awareness of communication skills can help the carer to become aware of the patient's condition. There may be further communication problems if the patient is non-English speaking, especially if there are also cultural problems; for example, Moslem women would be unhappy to see a male doctor. Help with communicating may be found for example:

- from the patient's relatives and friends
- by contacting the local Education Authority to

find out the name of the English as a Second Language (ESL) specialist who can help with interpreting

- by contacting the National Health Service
- by contacting the local Social Services Department
- by contacting the local branch of the Red Cross Society who have language cards written in the patient's native tongue

Deaf and blind patients need special consideration too. The elderly deaf patient may have lost his/her hearing fairly recently and may be finding it difficult to cope. The carer should take a few practical steps to help the patient. These include:

- speaking clearly, facing the patient so they can lip read and making regular eye contact
- using a low voice when talking (low frequencies are more easily heard by the partially deaf)

The blind or partially-sighted patient is unable to see non-verbal communication, so they will need plenty of verbal reassurance and explanations of what is happening around them as well as body contact. In old age, there may be difficulty in hearing too. The carer therefore needs to be especially considerate of the patient's needs.

Administering drugs

Although the patient's medical condition will be monitored by a doctor and district nurse, any drugs prescribed and any other treatment given will often have to be administered by the home carer. Most drugs are potentially dangerous so the right dose should always be given and the correct method used and the drugs should be administered to the patient at the time stated on the label. Drugs should never be given to someone else, and a doctor should always be consulted before the patient is given drugs which have been bought over the counter. The major point to make is that it is important that the label on any form of drug is read to check that it is the correct drug and that the drug is being given to the correct patient.

1. *Pills, capsules and tablets* These should be swallowed with a mouthful of water. If the patient finds this difficult, the pills, capsules or tablets can be crushed and taken in a spoonful of jam or honey.

2. *Powders* Again, they can be mixed with jam or honey or taken in a small glass of water, fruit juice or milk.

3. *Liquid medicines* The bottle should be shaken before opening, and the correct measure given on a medicine spoon or in a measuring glass. The medicine should be stored as instructed on the bottle.

4. *Suppositories* These are drugs that are pushed up into the rectum. The carer should wash her/his hands and ask the patient to lie on his/her side and try to relax. After putting on rubber gloves, the carer pushes the suppository up the rectum as far as his/her finger will reach.

5. *Inhalations* Inhalent drugs are either added to hot water and the steam breathed in, or they come in the form of an aerosol spray that the patient can use for themselves.

6. *Eardrops* The patient needs to put his/her head sideways on to a flat surface so the infected ear is uppermost. The carer should hold the filled dropper as close to the ear as possible and gently squeeze the dropper so the drops may be counted as they go into the ear. The patient needs to stay in the same position for a minute or two to ensure that the drops have reached the middle ear.

7. *Eyedrops* If possible, the carer should stand behind the patient to give eyedrops. The lower eyelid should be pulled down carefully and gently with the hand holding the dropper and the head should be steadied with the other hand. The dropper should be held horizontally, squeezed carefully, and the number of drops counted. The patient should then close his/her eyes and blink a few times to spread the drops over the eyeball.

8. *Nosedrops* Nosedrops should be given with the patient's head tilted back. The dropper is put just inside the nostril so the number of drops can be counted. As with eardrops, the patient should stay in the same position for a minute or two while the drops are sniffed up into the nasal passages.

9. *Medicines applied directly to the skin* These include creams, lotions, ointments, powders, pastes and liniments and should be applied as instructed.

10. *Injections* These will usually be given by a doctor or district nurse.

11. *Pessaries* These are drugs which are administered by being pushed up into the vagina. They are best given before the patient sleeps as there will be less physical movement taking place.

There are some general guidelines about administering drugs which include the following:

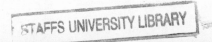
STAFFS UNIVERSITY LIBRARY

- the course of drugs should always be completed if it states so on the label
- any side-effects should be reported to a doctor immediately
- any left-over drugs should be thrown away by flushing them down the toilet to avoid them being taken in error
- the instructions on the label should always be followed; a stronger dose should never be given
- drugs should be locked away out of the reach of the patient and children

Nursing care of the elderly in hospital

Everything that has been covered in the previous section on home nursing applies to nursing the elderly in hospital, with the exception that hospital nurses are qualified and nurse as a profession. Hospital nurses, however, require the same qualities of patience and understanding, and they still need to put the patients first. Many of the duties they carry out in the course of the day require specialised nurse training and will not be carried out by a home nurse. They will also have more patients to care for, so their time will be more limited.

Nowadays, nursing the elderly patient is as likely to take place in medical and surgical wards as in a specialised care of the elderly unit. Nurses are aware of the need to treat the patient, not just the symptoms, and nursing the elderly is no longer seen to be inferior.

The nurse caring for an elderly patient will be encouraged to help the patient maintain his/her dignity by allowing them as much privacy as possible in, for example, the following situations:

- when washing and dressing
- when going to the toilet
- when being examined
- if incontinent
- if discussing a personal problem

The patient is still an individual, even though they are one of many on a ward. Good wards will allow the patients to maintain as much individuality as possible. Patients may be allowed to sleep in their own nightclothes, have personal effects in their bedside lockers, have a choice of meals, go to bed when they want to and so on. Independence needs to be encouraged, as in home nursing. Independence may, however, be more difficult on a practical basis in the ward as nursing staff change shifts and the new shift may not be aware of what the patient can and cannot do for him/herself. This emphasises the need for good record keeping to ensure that no

patients take a backward step. The hospital nurse will also need to deal with the patient's family on a number of different levels. When visiting the patient in hospital, they will ask the nurse for a progress report. If the patient is deteriorating and/or likely to die, the nurse needs to deal with the situation with tact and diplomacy.

- If the patient needs to continue treatment at home, after they have had an operation for example, the family will need to be educated so that they are able to deal with the situation.
- The relatives may need to know more about the patient's illness in order to understand certain changes in his/her lifestyle. For example, diabetics may need insulin injections, stroke patients will need physiotherapy, and so on.

When the nurse meets the relatives she/he has to make a fairly quick assessment of them: whether they are sympathetic, whether they can understand the information he/she is giving them, whether they will be able to help with the treatment at home. This demands certain skills that will develop with experience. Medical care of the elderly is based on teamwork in a hospital, no one person is wholly responsible for the patient's care. The different professionals who work in a hospital are described on page 36. The nurse is part of this team and is the person who is in contact with the patient the most. This means that the nurse will need to explain the role of the team to the patient and also be able to work with the other people in the team. In many cases she/he will be working as part of a multidisciplinary team (for example, with a stroke patient, the nurse may have to work with a doctor, a physiotherapist and an occupational therapist).

Summary of keypoints

- The patient's medical, emotional, physical and social needs should be the major consideration of the carer. These needs are constantly changing and need frequent reassessment.
- Home nursing has the advantage of offering the patient familiar surroundings and a known carer with whom they can communicate more freely.
- Consultation with professional agencies such as a health visitor, district nurse, doctor and social worker is important in order to work out whether home nursing is a viable possibility and to plan the input of the support services.
- The carer needs to consider carefully the demands that will be made on her/him.

Counselling should be available to her/him to outline and support them in their role as carer.

- The amount of care given to the patient needs to be carefully monitored: too much care and the patient becomes overdependent; too little care and the patient's rate of recovery can be affected.
- Everyday personal hygiene can help speed up the process of recovery as the patient will feel cleaner and more comfortable and be less likely to develop infections.
- Effective communication between carer and patient is vital, especially as the patient may find that communication becomes more difficult due to the nature of their illness.
- Professional nurses still need the same qualities of patience and understanding as the home carer. Their time will, however, be limited as they will have more than one patient to care for and there will be various nurses caring for the patient as shift changes occur.

Assignments

1. Think about the qualities needed to nurse an elderly patient. Do they differ if the nurse is a professional or a member of the family? Compile a set of guidelines on good nursing.

2. List the advantages and disadvantages of home nursing and hospital nursing. Include the needs of the patient and carer.

3. Suggest ways of promoting dignity and privacy in the everyday care of an elderly patient who is being nursed at home.

4. Discuss the reasons why some people may not be able to nurse an elderly patient.

5. As a group, discuss how respect for the patient can be incorporated into home and professional nursing.

6. Sometimes the stress caused by nursing can put the carer into the situation where they may hit their elderly relative. What are the danger signs to look for that may show that the carer is reaching the end of their tether? What help and advice might they be given?

7. Design a sick room for the elderly, immobile patient being cared for in the average home.

8. The daily care routine of the elderly patient depends on the seriousness of their illness. Look at the patient–care situations below and make some brief suggestions for a daily routine that incorporates the following patient needs:

- personal hygiene
- cleaning the sick room
- eating and drinking
- social
- emotional
- medical

The patients.

- A 75-year-old grandmother, staying at her son and daughter-in-law's house while she recovers from a mild bout of acute bronchitis. The doctor has recommended the following treatment:
  (i) bedrest in an upright position
  (ii) a light diet with plenty of fluids
  (iii) a course of antibiotics and painkillers
  (iv) a warm environment
- An 84-year-old grandfather staying at his daughter and son-in-law's house. He has been discharged from hospital with terminal cancer and needs a great deal of home nursing. The doctor has recommended the following treatment:
  (i) a district nurse to visit regularly throughout the day and night to administer painkillers and for continence management
  (ii) helping the patient to keep in touch with the life of the family and be emotionally supported
  (iii) eating a very light diet

9. Bed making looks complicated but becomes easier with practice. Practise making a bed with and without a patient in it. Use both blankets and a duvet.

10. Invite a district nurse or nurse to demonstrate to your group how to do the following home nursing tasks:

- bed making
- bed bathing
- moving and lifting a patient
- using a bedpan or urinal

11. The carer may be required to carry out various tests in the home. Ask a district nurse to explain and/or demonstrate some of the following tests:

- collecting urine, sputum, faecal and vomit samples. Ask how they are collected, how they are analysed and the disorders they might disclose

- faecal observation, i.e., what changes in the stools may suggest
- recording fluid input and output, i.e., measuring the amount of fluid taken in by the patient and the amount lost by urinating, diarrhoea, sweating or vomiting

12.   As a group, set aside some time for a practical session where the following nursing tasks can be practised:

- bed making with a patient in bed
- bed bathing, including hair washing
- moving and lifting a patient, including giving a bedpan
- feeding a patient in bed
- taking temperature, pulse and respiration

13.   Find out about the services available in your local area to cater for people whose first language is not English. Check whether there is any provision for interpreting their needs as patients.

14.   Drugs are carefully labelled by a pharmacist to help ensure that patients take the correct dose at the correct time. Find out about the labelling of drugs by personal research or by asking a local pharmacist to come and talk to your group. Find out about the correct storage and disposal of drugs. A pharmacist may also be able to help with assignment 15.

15.   Find out when and why the following drugs and treatments may be used:

- enema
- pessary
- suppository
- antibiotic
- ointment
- nosedrops
- eyedrops
- an inhalant

16.   Try and arrange a visit to your local hospital care of the elderly unit to find out about the day-to-day nursing care of the elderly. Speak to both nurses and patients.

17.   It is very easy to 'talk down' to the elderly which can be patronising and degrading to the patient. Discuss a set of guidelines that the carer could follow in order to build up a good relationship with the patient.

06188757

LIST OF USEFUL ADDRESSES

Age Concern England
Bernard Sunley House
60 Pitcairn Road
Mitcham
Surrey CR4 3LL

Alcohol Concern
305 Grays Inn Road
London WC1X 8QF

Alzheimer's Disease Society
158/160 Balham High Road
London SW12 9BN

Arthritis Care
6 Grosvenor Crescent
London SW1X 7ER

British Deaf Association
38 Victoria Place
Carlisle
Cumbria CA1 1HU

British Pensioners and Trades Union Action
Association
Norman Dodds House
315 Bexley Road
North Heath
Erith
Kent

Carers National Association
29 Chilworth Mews
London W2 3RG

Chest, Heart & Stroke Association
Tavistock House North
Tavistock Square
London WC1H 9JE

CRUSE, The National Organisation for the
Widowed & their Children
Cruse House
126 Sheen Road
Richmond
Surrey TW9 1UR

Disabled Living Foundation
380–384 Harrow Road
London W9 2HU

Help the Aged
St James's Walk
London EC1R OBE

MIND
National Association for Mental Health
22 Harley Street
London W1N 2ED

Pre-Retirement Association
19 Undine Street
Tooting
London SW17 8PP

Royal National Institute for the Blind
224 Great Portland Street
London W1N 6AA

Voluntary Euthanasia Society
13 Prince of Wales Terrace
London W8 5PG

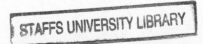
STAFFS UNIVERSITY LIBRARY

INDEX